"This is a treasure of practical wisdom. Knowing that exercise is good for you doesn't always translate to knowing how to get moving and stay moving in your own exercise program. Kate Hays talks plainly about how to do it! I highly recommend this book."

—Michael J. Mahoney, Ph.D., Professor of Psychology, University of North Texas and author of *Human Change Processes*

THE WORKOUT THERAPY WORKBOOK

MOVE
YOUR BODY
TONE
YOUR MOOD

A SCIENTIFICALLY PROVEN PROGRAM TO HELP
YOU EASE ANXIETY, LIFT DEPRESSION,
MANAGE STRESS, AND ENJOY YOUR BODY

KATE F. HAYS, PH.D.

NEW HARBINGER PUBLICATIONS, INC.

Distributed in the U.S.A. by Publishers Group West; in Canada by Raincoast Books; in Great Britain by Airlift Book Company, Ltd.; in South Africa by Real Books, Ltd.; in Australia by Boobook; and in New Zealand by Tandem Press.

Copyright © 2002 by Kate F. Hays
New Harbinger Publications, Inc.
5674 Shattuck Avenue
Oakland, CA 94609

Cover design by Salmon Studios
Edited by Carole Honeychurch
Cover and interior illustrations by Stephanie Carter/Artville
Book design by Michele Waters

ISBN 1-57224-275-2 Paperback

New Harbinger Publications' Web site address: www.newharbinger.com

04   03   02

10   9   8   7   6   5   4   3   2   1

First printing

To my guys, JEB and EHL, who lead, follow, and stand with me in equal measure.

CONTENTS

Part 1
"But I Thought Therapy Was All Talk!"
How Exercise Can Be Your Therapy

Part 2
How to Be Therapeutic to Yourself Through Exercise

Part 3
"Now What?" Maintaining Your Gains

Part 4
Taking a "Fearless Inventory": Review and Reflection

"BUT I THOUGHT THERAPY WAS ALL TALK!" HOW EXERCISE CAN BE YOUR THERAPY

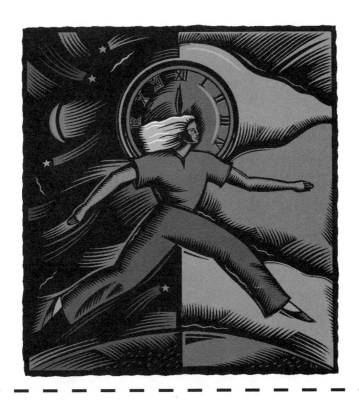

Chapter 1

An Introduction: Starting on Your Path

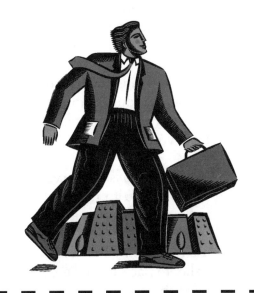

Welcome to this workbook and our journey together. This book is designed to take you down some well-worn paths and show you many new vistas. Some of our travels will involve new territory or unfamiliar footing. My hope is that you will find this adventure interesting, informative, and action-inspiring.

Your journey will be most meaningful to you if you take two actions right away. One of these is adopting an attitude: thinking of yourself as an investigator or a searcher for truth. The other action is making a commitment to one form of sedentary activity: writing out your thoughts.

The Scientist or Detective Approach

An attitude of curiosity or experimentation is vital to beginning and continuing this exercise adventure. It might help to think of yourself as a scientist. For our purposes, you can be Marie Curie, experimenting with different hypotheses and having the opportunity to put them to the test. Or you could picture yourself as a detective—Sherlock Holmes looking for clues in your behavior to solve the mystery of you and your relationship to physical activity. This kind of investigative approach is useful in a number of ways. Being inquisitive will help maintain your interest. And if you have some mental-health concerns, this attitude of curiosity can counteract the hopelessness of depression or the tension of anxiety. Further, this perspective allows you to be more objective. You'll notice the effects of exercise and come to trust your experience. Exercise and exercise effects are behaviorally measurable and thus provide an excellent opportunity for you to be that scientist or detective with yourself.

Journaling

People keep journals for many reasons. One of these is to get a clearer perspective on yourself. Journals allow you to be both subject and object, making statements to yourself about yourself. A journal is a place for reflection rather than a place of judgment. Keeping a journal also allows you to individualize and adapt *Move Your Body . . .* to your needs and interests, so that what you are reading becomes directly applicable to your unique life. As you develop your new exercise skills, your "scientist self" can use your journal to state and explore hypotheses, discovering new vistas. Your "detective self" can use the journal to find relevant clues.

Recording your thoughts allows you to find out what you think. A journal is a place where you can:

Make observations. Observations can take a variety of forms. Some of the Journal Tasks encourage you to notice your feelings and behaviors and reflect on what you discover. At other times, you may incorporate your observations into your ongoing Exercise Log.

Make commitments to yourself. Because you are in dialogue with yourself, a journal is an excellent space to make commitments to yourself about who you want to be and how you wish to act.

Review what you're actually doing. Once scientists have conducted their experiments, they observe the results. Detectives pull together various clues to form their working assessment. In the same way, your journal will become a storehouse of information about yourself, allowing you to have a specific place where you can gather the results and draw conclusions. Your journal is a vehicle for you to be able to review yourself rather than mis-remember—or not remember at all.

Revise and reassess your plan. Scientists revise their working hypotheses based on the results of their experiments, and detectives synthesize their information to see if there are facts for which they have yet to account. Because a journal is an ongoing process and because it's for your eyes only, you can use your journal to revise and reassess what you are doing.

Keeping Track

Throughout this book you will find sections marked "Exercise." These are short assignments designed for you to complete in the workbook. They give you the opportunity to personalize and reflect upon what you're reading. In addition to the Exercises, I have suggested a number of "Journal Tasks." These activities differ from the Exercises in that they are longer, more complex, or reflective. For these Journal Tasks, I'd encourage you to use a journal.

Journals vs. Diaries vs. Logs

What's the difference between a journal, a diary, and a log? Both "journal" and "diary" derive from Romance words referring to daily events. Traditionally, journals or diaries have been kept on a daily basis. I would encourage you to use your journal with the frequency that works best for you. Better to write meaningfully in your journal twice a week than to be daily diligent for a week and then stop altogether.

Your journal can take whatever form works best for you. In this book, you will see various suggestions. Some people like to use a bound volume. Others prefer looseleaf pages. Your computer may be the recipient for all your thoughts, to be sorted later. Experiment and find out what suits you best.

Some people like to stay right on task. Others find it interesting and informative to write more extensively. Intriguingly (we'll talk about this more in chapter 8), a journal kept specifically to record your thoughts or feelings while you were exercising may help you become aware of your fleeting but profound insights, similar to the kind you might notice during the early morning awakening time. Random thoughts, poetic phrases, special insights, and even new ways to organize a project or a meeting may all be more accessible during or shortly after exercise. This form of review adds its own level of richness to exercise.

The term "log" implies keeping a regular record. It may focus on activities rather than thoughts and feelings. I have reserved that term for your Exercise Log.

What Are the Rules of Journaling?

As someone who has kept journals for years and helped other people do so, too, there are only a few basic rules that I'd suggest you follow:

- Date everything that you write; because you're in the process of change, you will understand more about yourself if you know when you made which observations.

- Give yourself permission to write freely. A journal is a place where you *don't* need to pay attention to grammar or penmanship. Your journal is for you only.

- Have fun with your journal. Be creative. Sometimes using only words will do. Other times, you can express more through drawing, even if it's stick figures or symbols.

- If you feel self-conscious, write in the third person: "After one week of brisk walking, Janet found herself thinking more clearly."

Where Are We Going?

Let me give you a preliminary map of this internal and external exploration. In this first section, we'll focus on the "whys" and the "whats" of the mental benefits of exercise. You may or may not want to begin with these rationales and justifications. Chapter 4, "Designing Your Exercise Plan," however is a "must read" section of the book, since it's applicable to everyone.

In part 2, we'll look in depth at four specific ways that exercise is therapeutic: in regard to stress and anxiety, depression, self-esteem, and thinking. You may find one or more of these chapters especially relevant to you and your circumstances.

As you will come to appreciate, this exercise process is a journey for life. Part 3 examines some of the particulars of maintaining physical activity in a mentally healthy way. And finally, in part 4 we will put exercise together *with* psychotherapy in a variety of ways.

Now it's time to begin—time to start making sense of the body-mind connection in a new way. I won't say "sit back and relax." How about "step forward and relax"?

CHAPTER 2

Why Exercise Is Good for Your Head as Well as Your Heart

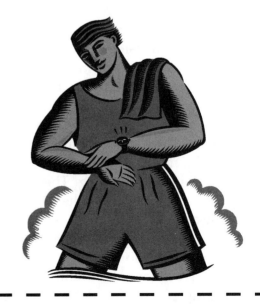

Suppose you could take a magic pill that would make you feel happy if you were sad, settle you down if you were stressed, calm your fears, and increase your self-esteem. Oh, and you would be more creative. Since, like most people, you care about how you look, you'd be pleased that this pill was able to determine and maintain your "just right" weight. And furthermore, people would comment on your appearance, saying that you just seemed younger, stronger, livelier. All this from one pill! And a pill with a low risk of negative side effects and few disadvantages.

These changes in your thoughts, feelings, attitudes, and appearance would be additional to all the physical effects of this pill, such as improving the functioning of your heart and your lungs and decreasing the risk of many chronic diseases.

"Let's have at it," you say.

Well, of course I'm describing exercise.

There is one major complicating factor: You have to be active in order to obtain these effects. Unlike the passive, low demand act of swallowing a pill, *you* have to get moving, choose what you're going to do, and then continue the process. Although it won't cost a lot in terms of money, you will need to invest—developing a plan will take thinking and preparation. And doing the activity will also take time.

The payoffs, however, are great. Carol and Mitchell Krucoff, authors of *Healing Moves*, sum them up nicely: "Getting regular physical activity may be *the single most important thing* you can do to prevent disease and promote good health" (emphasis added) (2000, p. 2). Your changed attitude about yourself will be an additional benefit. Because you're the person in charge, you will experience yourself as someone who is capable of having direct impact on your thoughts and feelings—your mental as well as physical well-being—through your own actions.

What Exercise Does to Your Mind as Well as Your Body

Perhaps you are not someone who exercises. You ask yourself: "Why would *anyone* do it?" Your doubts seem confirmed as you notice people in your daily life: you see a runner along the side of the road, sweating and grimacing, or a bicycle rider straining to get up a steep hill. Contrast these effortful or even unpleasant images you've seen with these people's report of their own feelings. Ask the runner, "Why do you run?" and her face will light up. She will probably say that running feels good and raises her spirits. The cyclist, too, will say that when he got to the top of that hill, he felt on top of the world. Now, part of that feeling is certainly a sense of accomplishment. And part of the feeling may be "Phew! It's done!" But these people will tell you that it goes beyond just the doing of the thing. There's a physical and psychological change that takes place in exercising people's bodies that goes by the technical term "the feel good" effect. Just as a sense of well-being is not merely the absence of ill health, feeling good is not only the opposite of depression. Feeling good involves a sense of zest and pleasure, a positive appreciation for life.

We know about and can often name the many physical benefits of exercise. For example, exercise decreases the risk of coronary heart disease and stroke while improving rehabilitative potential in both these conditions. Exercise impacts various coronary risk factors, including high blood pressure, cholesterol level and type, smoking, and obesity. It also decreases the risk of colon cancer and results in reduced body fat (or reduced total body mass and fat weight), lowered blood pressure, and improved carbohydrate metabolism. Exercise is associated with reduced problems or delay of problems related to diabetes, assists in the maintenance of bone density, helps improve the quality and quantity of sleep, creates increased oxygen capacity, and improves the functioning of your immune system. At least thirty-five health conditions are directly affected by your level of activity (Booth 2001; Crandall 1986; McDonald and Hodgdon 1991; United States Department of Health and Human Services 1996).

Even though just about anybody who exercises regularly will tell you that they feel better with exercise, the psychological benefits of exercise aren't as well known to the general public as are the physical effects. The connection between our minds and bodies is such an interactive and interconnected experience that there is a seamless loop relating to feeling good. Instead of "body" and "mind" as two separate entities, it's more like "bodymind" or "mindbody." In Western languages, we don't have one single word that can reflect this thought. Even in German, which often uses a single word to describe something that in English has many, we can only limp in with "Leib-Seele-Einheheit" or "body-mind-unity." But Eastern thought can help us out. The word "yoga" means "unity." And the Zen state of *satori* is the union of body, mind, and spirit.

We can think of this interaction as a spiral, where one turn leads to the next. For example, optimistic people tend to have better health than those who are pessimistic (Seligman 1991). This ties in directly with the effect of your mind on your body: if you feel positive, you will be healthier. And exercise can help in this chain reaction, as physical activity can affect your perspective of the world. Exercise and sport can tap into and enhance your sense of well-being, calmness, control, and attention to the present. And in fact, highly active people tend to be more optimistic and less pessimistic than those who are inactive (Kavussanu and McAuley 1995).

The Body-Mind Connection Is Not New News

Many centuries ago, Greek philosophers understood this positive connection between what we do with our bodies and how we feel. During the "Golden Age of Greece," much of the day involved vigorous physical activity for everyone—children, adults, and the elderly. This activity was conducted deliberately for its contribution toward mental as well as physical well-being (Seraganian 1993). Hippocrates is reported to have prescribed exercise for patients with mental illness. Aristotle saw happiness as the supreme good, with everything else in people's lives a means to this end. Or think of the classic phrase that Homer first spoke: "A healthy mind in a healthy body." (He said it in Greek, naturally, and Juvenal then translated it into Latin: "Mens sana in corpore sano.")

The Declaration of Independence recognized three inalienable, or basic and essential, rights. Perhaps the most intriguing one is "the pursuit of happiness." What does that mean? The pursuit of happiness is closely linked with your experience of the quality of your life. Researchers studying people's sense of subjective well-being or happiness recognize that this feeling includes the absence of negative mood, the presence of positive feelings, and high levels of life satisfaction (Diener 2000). And how does exercise relate to this? Exercise can have direct influence on your mood, your perception of stress, your physical health, and your sense of life satisfaction (Berger and Motl 2001). That's a pretty direct prescription for quality of life.

EXERCISE: New News

There are nearly daily reports about the relationship between exercise and well-being. Over the next week, as you embark on this process of discovery about yourself in relation to exercise, notice the news reports—in your newspaper, on TV, on the Web—about the benefits of physical activity. They're all around you; all you need to do is pay attention. Looking for and accumulating this information serves two functions. Your "scientist self" or your "detective self" will have more data. In addition, the process of searching and collecting itself will give you motivation, confirmation, and reinforcement in your body-mind quest. Write down the date and title of each relevant news item you come across:

Date   **Title**

_____   _____

_____   _____

_____   _____

_____   _____

You may want to clip or print hard copies of articles and begin a file folder containing news, research, and tips on exercise and well-being.

As we have shifted from an agrarian economy to increasingly sedentary occupations, physical activity has disappeared from the daily landscape of our lives. In 1900, "almost all of us died of infectious acute diseases. . . . Today nearly all of us will die from chronic diseases. . . . Chronic diseases are not simply the *natural consequence of aging*. They appear, in large part, to be the consequence of an *unnatural lifestyle*" [sic] (Johnsgard 1989, p. 16).

What was a part of our everyday lives, being physically active, has now shifted to something that is *un*natural. As if we had planned it, we are engineering inactivity and obesity into our culture. On average, we use 800 fewer calories per day than our parents did (Krucoff and Krucoff 2000).

Many of us have an image of our own energy as if it were a fixed and limited amount. Use up 10 percent and you only have 90 percent left for the day. Ironically, our attempts to conserve our energy backfire on us. Reducing energy expenditure leaves us more, rather than less, depleted.

-- -- -- -- -- -- -- -- -- -- -- -- -- -- -- -- -- -- -- --

EXERCISE: ENERGY DEPLETION

Here's another observation exercise to do, before you change anything. Over the next week, notice the obvious and subtle ways in which you save energy by limiting your activity. As we will discuss later, using energy in fact gives you energy. But many of us use any excuse to avoid expending energy "unnecessarily." What are some of the ways you opted out?

Date	Opportunity to use energy:	What I did instead:
5/28	Walking up and down 1 flight of stairs	Took elevator
5/30	Manually opening heavy outer door	Activating electronic opener
5/31	Walking into gas station to pay	Paying at the pump

-- -- -- -- -- -- -- -- -- -- -- -- -- -- -- -- -- -- -- --

JOURNAL TASK: ENERGY GENERATION

In your journal, start a page on increased daily activity. This page serves as a record for you of ways in which you are putting activity *into* your life. As with the examples above, it may be a very small or subtle change—but it signals a change in attention and attitude, as well as behavior.

Date   **Activity**

_____   _____

_____   _____

_____   _____

_____   _____

_____   _____

Now that we have increased physical leisure, exercise has become a task, sometimes seeming like a chore, that is supposed to be added into the day. When exercise is separated from the rest of our lives, it becomes foreign, effortful, and a burden. Rather than serving to integrate our body and mind, exercise that is viewed as a task or demand *dis*integrates who and what we are. As a culture, we have developed myths that keep us separate from exercise. Let's look at five of these myths.

Five Exercise Myths—and Truths

In our current society, the idea of exercise often takes on its own oppressive weight. Exercise can be viewed as obligatory, compulsory, effortful, anti-leisure, and unnatural. Alternatively, we can view exercise as actively chosen, fun or playful, energy-adding, active, and natural.

Obligation vs. Choice

When exercise is viewed as obligatory, it becomes another chore, another "should." Instead, we might think of physical activity as central to being human. Dr. George Sheehan, dubbed the "philosopher king" of running by Bill Clinton, quoted another philosopher, Bertrand Russell, to bolster his argument about the pivotal nature of exercise to our being: "'Man is an animal, and his happiness depends on his physiology more than he likes to think. . . . Unhappy businessmen would increase their happiness more by walking six miles every day than by any conceivable change in philosophy'" (1996, p. 48).

Compulsory vs. Fun

When activity feels compulsory, the fun and pleasure that help sustain it are instead drained out. Routine becomes flat rather than reassuringly predictable. Excuses are found. Our basic mental and physical satisfaction lose their luster. In an extended riff on the playfulness of exercise, Sheehan described three fundamental functions of play:

> Play is essential to the good life. We need it to become fully functioning human beings. . . . The first influence of play is on our bodies. It brings with it exercise. Medicine and surgery attack disease but they do not cover health. That resides in the fully functioning body, be it sick or well. Health is the best we can be. Health is getting the most out of the body we were born with. The playful use of the exercising body is what brings this about.
>
> The second influence of play is on our attitude. It encourages a sense of humor. . . . Humor allows us to be serious while having the feeling that it is all a game. Or we can come to a project knowing it is a game yet realizing how serious that game is.
>
> The final effect of play is on our conduct. . . . We must learn from ourselves. We must trust the inner person. The experiences in play are immediate, graphic, and illuminating. We learn the fundamental characteristics of our own personal human nature. In play we reveal ourselves—to others as well as to ourselves. Play is an unrivaled area for self-discovery. (1996, p. 62f)

The cartoon strip "Cathy" illustrates the contrast between child and adult experiences of exercise: a delighted child runs among playground equipment in a picture entitled "The Gym, Ages 1-10." In contrast, "The Gym, Rest of Life," shows Cathy in anxious tears as she stands at the door of a fitness center. A large sign is posted: "New Thigh Machines." In the six pictures that follow, Cathy and a friend watch her friend's young daughter run, go up and down steps, lift buckets of sand, ride her bike, and then beg to go swimming. Observing her, the two adults discuss the work that they have created of exercise. Plaintively they ask: "Why can't it still be fun for us?"

Research backs up this observation: when children are involved in youth sports, intrinsic factors, such as fun, accomplishment, challenge, improving skills, and excitement are the central factors of their enjoyment. And when adults experience exercise as fun, they don't have difficulty motivating themselves to get out and "just do it."

Physician Joan Ullyot described the ways in which she became aware of the pleasure of activity. She also described the contrast between her own approach and that of her husband. (These gender-based observations of twenty-five years ago still seem to have some validity today.)

> Even for those who have run before, this feeling [the joy of movement] may be new. In my first years of running, my husband, a 440–yard dash specialist in high school, couldn't understand why I ran. I tried to explain. . . .
>
> He frowned and cross-examined me. "Let me get this straight, Joan. Do you mean to say you actually get some sort of *physical pleasure* out of running?"

Blushing and feeling as if I were confessing some perversion, I admitted to it.

"Then you're not doing it right," he snapped. "You have to run harder!"

That, I have since learned, is the typical advice of the 440 runner for whom training is agony and the only reward is faster times. It took weeks of enjoyable, aerobically paced running with me ("Do you always run this slow?" he would ask) to convert him to the pleasure principle (Ullyot 1976, p. 11).

Effortful vs. Energy-Additive

Most of us have decided that activity is effortful. But in fact, activity *creates* energy. When you're tired, a walk around the block will help wake you up and feel energy for the task that seemed exhausting or insurmountable a few minutes before.

Sedentary vs. Active

Our image of leisure time means *in*action: What comes to mind when you think of leisure? Perhaps lolling on the beach or being transported on a carriage ride. There's even the proverbial joke about eating bonbons while watching TV. Yet in a way, that type of leisure can actually feel exhausting and paralyzing. This perspective on leisure can be compared to the ancient Chinese custom of foot binding. Rather than becoming liberated to take pleasure in their leisure, these upper-class women's bodies were disfigured and their lives constricted by the demands of class and gender. Similarly, the "privilege" of sedentary repose could be robbing us of our vitality.

Unnatural vs. Natural

If activity is understood as unnatural and not part of everyday life, it makes sense to assume that occasional or sporadic activity will be sufficient. After a brief stint, you've met your obligation. Let's challenge this assumption by applying it to other natural aspects of our being. For example, do you object to sleep at night? Do you plan to stock up on sleep so that you won't need to do it again? Do you say, "If I get eight hours of sleep for two weeks, then I'll be perfectly rested for the next three months"?

These absurdly rhetorical questions obviously demand "no" for an answer. We haven't yet programmed out of our bodies the need for sleep. Sometimes we play around the edges. We may get to bed late, drag ourselves up to the sound of an alarm, and use coffee to get us going in the morning—when what we really need is two more hours of sleep. The same can be said for our need for movement. Being human involves meeting certain essential needs, such as eating, sleeping—and moving. "Regular exercise is required to fulfill our genetic design specifications for normal, trouble-free functioning" (Johnsgaard 1989, p. 23).

Of course, as with sleep, we need some regularity of activity in order for it to be beneficial. The phrase "use it or lose it" applies to the mental benefits of exercise as much as to any other habit. A study of 944 elderly men and women who exercised at least three times a week found that most were not depressed. When surveyed again five years later, those still exercising regularly continued to be free of depression, while those who were no longer exercising scored similarly to people who had not been exercising all along. The good news is that it's really never too late: a group who had not been exercising during the first study but began before the follow-up also showed the nondepressed scores (Kritz-Silverstein, Barrett-Connor, and Corbeau 2001).

EXERCISE: EXERCISE MYTHS

What exercise myths do you bring to this discussion? Can you identify some beliefs that hold you back from activity?

The Exercise Gateway

Our focus on health and disease has shifted, especially during the past century. The first health-care revolution was intended to wipe out infectious diseases. The mortality rate changed dramatically with the various discoveries and changes in practice around sanitation, immunization, and vaccination against pandemic disease. The second revolution focused on eliminating degenerative diseases, and indeed, increased longevity has resulted. The third revolution—the one we're still in the midst of—attends to health and wellness as compared with disease. Prevention is vital, and active consumer involvement drives the engine of this revolution. Self-help is the keyword. The health and mental health benefits of physical activity are a central aspect of this phase. A parallel in the mental health field can be seen in the new positive psychology. "The field of positive psychology . . . is about valued subjective experiences: well-being, contentment, and satisfaction (in the past); hope and optimism (for the future); and flow and happiness (in the present)" (Seligman and Csikszentmihalyi 2000, p. 5).

It is intriguing and hopeful that changing your health habits can start anywhere. These habit changes will all—if you let them—"speak" to you and help guide you toward what works best for your particular body. I'm suggesting starting with exercise, because often, without you doing anything else, physical activity assists you in beginning to take better care of your overall health. For that reason, exercise is called a

EXERCISE: YOUR HEALTH GATEWAY

What is your health gateway? Is your gate smoothly oiled and able to swing freely, or is it creaky and rusty?

Below are a number of health habits that help us function well. Are you already engaged in some of them? If so, put a check mark next to them. If not, place a zero.

Nutritious eating   _____

Weight under control   _____

Sufficient sleep (seven to eight hours)   _____

Regular exercise   _____

Not smoking   _____

No or minimal alcohol   _____

Below, draw your own links among these behaviors. Which are connected to which for you? What will need to change?

For example, you might be aware that when you get enough sleep, the food that you consume is more nutritionally balanced and, in turn, you stay at a more stable weight. Your links would look like this:

Sufficient sleep ——→Nutritious eating ——→Stable weight

Or exercise may help you recognize actual physical hunger and may also have impact on your weight. Eating appropriately may in turn help you regulate alcohol consumption. Exercise may help you feel sufficiently tired at night so that you sleep deeply. Your gateway would be linked like this:

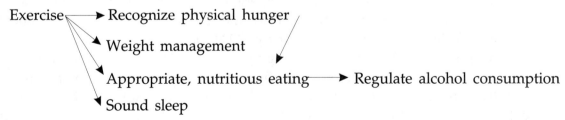

"gateway" behavior: if you walk through the exercise "gate," you are likely to develop other healthy habits of life. You will eat more appropriately, sleep will feel deeper and better, cigarette smoking will lose its appeal—there's even talk that sex is improved. Repeatedly, research finds that exercise is associated with improved health habits in general (Crandall 1986; McDonald and Hodgdon 1991; United States Department of Health and Human Services 1996). A "virtuous" rather than a "vicious" cycle has thus been established, in which one aspect of being healthy supports another that creates another. You do good, feel good, look good, and think good.

Why Exercise Is Mentally Effective

A number of physiological and psychological hypotheses have been offered over the years to explain this intimate relationship between physical activity and mental health. At this point, there is no conclusive evidence that any of the explanations is *the* correct one. However, all are interesting. As you exercise and understand your own body-mind connection more completely, you may find that some seem particularly relevant to you.

Brain Chemicals

For the past twenty years, people have talked about the release of endorphins, chemical agents within our brains, to explain the positive mood that occurs with exercise. No doubt there's something to this hypothesis—although the reality is probably more complicated than it seems. Endorphins are brain chemicals similar to morphine, and like morphine and other opiates, they may trigger feelings of euphoria and tension relief and increase our pain tolerance. However, the measurement of brain endorphins is difficult, and so we don't yet know the exact biochemical changes.

In recent years, we've also recognized other important brain chemicals that may be responsible for some of the positive effects people experience from exercise. These other types of brain chemicals, or neurotransmitters, include monoamines such as serotonin, dopamine, and norepinephrine. (These brain chemicals may sound very familiar. The action of these neurotransmitters is the effective base for recently developed medications that decrease depression and anxiety, such as Prozac and other selective serotonin reuptake inhibitors, or SSRIs.) These neurotransmitters may have some of the same effects as endorphins, but exercise physiologists are more cautious about claiming this truth than is the popular press or the general public (Leith 1994; Morgan 1997).

EXERCISE: YOUR FEEL-GOOD EFFECT

When you are physically active, does it seem to you that something "just happens" and you start to feel happier or less tense? Under what conditions?

_____

_____

_____

The Thermogenic Hypothesis

This theory suggests that the elevation in your core body temperature, occurring during and after at least moderate exercise, influences your emotions. In particular, the increased warmth may account for a reduction in tension or anxiety. This is not unlike taking a bath, which can leave you feeling relaxed and calm. And certainly Scandinavians have regularly used sauna baths for both mental and physical well-being for over a thousand years. Yet, as you will see, some people experience mental benefits from physical activity even if they don't "work up a good sweat."

EXERCISE: WHEN YOU'RE HOT,
YOU'RE COOL

When you are physically active, can you feel yourself getting warmer all the way through your body? Does it seem like the warmth or the exertion helps change your mood? Is there an upper limit to the warmth that you find satisfying?

_____

_____

_____

_____

_____

Cognitive, Mental, and Psychological Hypotheses

Various psychological hypotheses have also been proposed concerning the mechanisms underlying mental well-being through physical activity. These psychological perspectives focus on how we think and feel. Distraction, self-esteem, and sociability are all possible explanations.

The "distraction" hypothesis suggests that exercise provides a legitimate "time-out" from our everyday preoccupations. Action provides distraction. *Doing* something else can allow us to *think* about something else.

People who exercise regularly have higher self-esteem and a greater general sense of accomplishment. While this may be something of a chicken and egg issue, a number of researchers have studied the increased sense of self-mastery, self-efficacy, and self-esteem that occurs with people who exercise. We'll discuss these positive effects in chapter 7.

The regulation of "social distance" may also be a relevant factor. For many people, the social interaction and engagement that occurs with certain forms of exercise—whether taking a class at a gym with others or being part of a team—may be the driving force in the pleasure of physical activity. And for others, the polar opposite is important: Exercise may be the occasion for a time of solitude and internal contemplation.

- -

EXERCISE: IT'S ALL IN YOUR HEAD

Which psychological aspects of physical activity are relevant for you? Do you think differently with exercise? Does exercise leave you feeling emotionally stronger? Is exercise most satisfying for you if it's with other people or if you have time to yourself?

_____

_____

_____

_____

_____

_____

_____

- -

Combinations and Interactions

Each of the above hypotheses may be accurate for some people, or to be even more specific, for some people in regard to certain kinds of exercise. Or a number of these effects may interact to provide the difference you feel after exercise. For example, raising your core body temperature may influence the release of certain mood-enhancing biochemicals in your brain. The increased relaxation and sense of comfort in your body may mean that you are less tense, more friendly, and have a natural topic of conversation in your interactions with others in the locker room. Or your increased sense of competence may influence your belief system, which in turn impacts your self-esteem. Being part of a group may change your perceptions and beliefs about yourself. And so on.

Forty-seven-year-old Rick is a triathlete and thus exercises by running, swimming, and cycling. (Throughout *Move Your Body, Tone Your Mind*, I will be sharing some stories with you. The people are quite real—they are friends, colleagues, and clients—but in all cases I've disguised enough details that people's privacy has been protected.) In part because of these different activities and in part because he is self-reflective and attentive, Rick's observations provide a powerful understanding of the many ways in which exercise can have impact on one's thoughts and relationships.

■ Rick's Story

When he works out on a track, Rick's focus is on technique and little else. The same is true for swimming. Because swimming is his weakest skill, most of the swim time is directed toward improving his technique and attempting to keep count of the laps. But with cycling, he finds much more flexibility. Some rides are long, social "conversation pace" rides with his training partner or his wife. Conversation is liable to be about anything: "We've used those rides to talk about issues in our lives. We've dealt with deaths, job changes, births of babies, or everyday dilemmas," Rick commented. Cycling with a "pack" of other people shifts the focus to time, distance, external events, and the sense of connection he feels with others who are also involved in the hard, sweaty, exhilarating work of an intense workout. And then there are long, slow distance runs that he takes as times for reflecting and planning

Rick commented: "On a day-to-day basis, regular exercise helps my cognitive processes. I think, plan, and execute tasks better. I enjoy the benefits of better health, improved stamina, and being able to do things that others my age may not. Exercise is also a major stress release. It helps me put things in perspective and balance. My wife has remarked on more than one occasion when I am ruminating over an irritation, 'Don't you need to go for a run?'"

As you read this book, you will come to understand that there is no one exercise that is "right" for everyone. As you become even more active in your own health care, you can become clearer about your own hypotheses: what is it about what kind of exercise, when, and how much works for you—and why.

Cautions and Pitfalls to Avoid

Although I am enthusiastic about the mental benefits of exercise and hope that you are, too (or will be soon), some cautions seem relevant before we embark on this process of discovery. These include:

- For some people, the mental changes will be nearly instantaneous. For others, it will be a matter of accumulated experience and activity or increased intensity that can only occur after you've reached a certain level of conditioning. Be curious and find out what is true for you.

- Exercising *does* involve lifestyle changes. These may be as simple as recognizing what you're going to do less of in order to make time for exercise. They may be as complex as changes in who's going to pick up the kids or when dinner is going to happen. You can anticipate and make plans about some of these alterations. You will notice others as they occur.

- If you tend to overdo things—people sometimes refer to this as an "addictive" personality—be aware that exercise can serve the same cluttering function as other activities. Exercise may help you feel better by helping you avoid the emotional issues that you really need to be paying attention to. We'll talk about this in some detail in chapters 10 and 11.

- Although exercise is an effective tool in stress management, it's not necessarily *more* effective than other stress-management techniques. Meditation, the relaxation response, progressive relaxation, and stress inoculation training can all be used to handle stress (Bahrke and Morgan 1978; Berger, Friedman, and Eaton 1988; Long 1985; Long and Haney 1988). You can change your mood through other methods, as well, whether prayer, listening to or making music, spending time with friends, or eating and drinking. In contrast to these other methods though, exercise has some distinguishing features—those health and physical appearance benefits we've already discussed. Exercise may also be different in the duration of its benefits and the patterns of mood change that it provides.

- No matter how persuasive I am or how much you know that exercise would be helpful to you, this may not be the moment in your life when you're going to make this particular change. Think about the differences in how children learn to walk. Oblivious to danger or risk, nine-month-old Sandra gets up, wobbles, walks a few steps, crashes, and eagerly picks herself up again. Sam, on the other hand, nearly a year older, still holds onto furniture or an outstretched hand, carefully assessing the situation—until the day when he just gets up and starts walking. If you're more like Sam than Sandra, sit back, relax, learn, and pay attention to why exercise won't work for you right now. All of these approaches will help you to just take off when you're ready.

- In this book, I am only speaking to you. You are interested in the body-mind question. You want to improve your mental health. But "you" may be someone with just a few everyday worries or you may be someone with a lot of complicated and difficult-to-resolve problems. Although I will be addressing the mental benefits of physical activity, it is very clear to me that for many people psychotherapy is an important tool to sorting out your life—whether psychotherapy alone or in conjunction with exercise. So, even though we'll only talk about psychotherapy at the end of the book (chapter 13), please consider psychotherapy if it seems appropriate to you.

Now that you've had a chance to consider the mental benefits of physical activity, perhaps you're ready to get started. In the next two chapters, we'll look at a number of aspects to starting to exercise: changing your habits, choosing the right exercise for you, and setting goals.

CHAPTER 3

"What's in It For Me?" Getting Started Doing Exercise

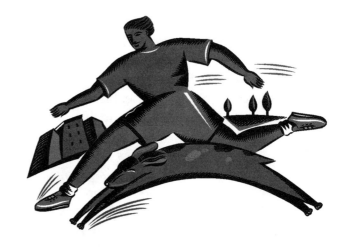

B efore plunging into the exercise waters, let's do some theory building so that you can understand how prepared you are to begin exercising and what you need to do to get ready. For any kind of change that you undertake, whether weight loss, smoking cessation, breast self-examination, or exercise, researchers have identified five steps essential to change (Prochaska, Norcross, and DiClemente 1994).

The Stage of Change Model

How do you go about changing patterns of behavior? Often, we think that change is like an "on/off" switch. First you aren't doing something, then you decide to change and voilà! You simply begin doing it. Let's use a nonexercise example to explore this approach. Suppose you decide you want to lose weight. You might assume that losing weight is just a matter of willpower, of deciding to go on a diet and lose those ten extra pounds. But actually, people are much more complicated than this "either/or" model suggests. In fact, this "just do it" perspective is really the fourth of five steps involved in change.

Change is a process. It takes conscious effort to shift long-standing habits. Let's start at the beginning, which is before you even begin thinking about change. The first stage of change is called "Precontemplation." Precontemplation is the stage during which other people around you may think you should do something, but you aren't even considering it. This time of rationalizing and discounting can take many forms. Using the weight-loss example, you might say to yourself, "I'm under too much stress," or "It's good to have some extra padding in winter," and so on. Stage two is known as "Contemplation," the time when you wonder about or contemplate a certain kind of change. At this point in your decision making about weight loss, for example, you're probably noticing that there seem to be a lot of media stories lately about lifestyle changes, or appropriate BMI (body-mass index) ratings. You start to think about other times you've attempted to lose weight and begin sorting out what was useful then.

As you become more comfortable with the idea of changing your behavior, you begin making changes. Not necessarily consistent changes or even the changes that you're ultimately shooting for. You may spend quite a while thinking about a change, trying it out, and going back and forth with it. In terms of weight loss, you might go on a drastic diet for a few days, and then fall off the wagon for the zillionth time. You might acknowledge that extreme deprivation isn't going to be successful in the long run. Perhaps you stock up on healthy foods that you like, getting yourself and your environment ready to embark on weight change. These small first steps help comprise stage three, or "Preparation."

And then it becomes clear: you've got a plan, you begin to stick to it regularly, and you notice the effects of this change, whether in terms of thoughts, feelings, or behavior. This is stage four, the "Action" stage. In the weight loss example, you're systematically noticing when you're truly hungry. You eat with intention and attention. You're limiting your intake of fat, using the nutritional food pyramid as a guide. You make plans about when and what to eat, and your actions are persistent and consistent.

But that's not the end of the progression. There's also stage five, because once you do change, it takes a while for this new behavior to become a habit. So the fifth stage is "Maintenance," which may be the most challenging stage of all. People who lose weight and are able to maintain that weight loss typically find that there are a whole range of lifestyle modifications that accompany this process, and it takes time and repetition to truly understand and make use of those alterations. (And a not so secret secret: Maintenance of weight loss involves regular exercise!)

The Stages of Change and Exercise

Researchers who have studied these stages have found consistent patterns regarding various changes in health behaviors. At any one time, about 40 percent of people are in the Precontemplation stage, about 40 percent are in the Contemplation or Preparation stages, and about 20 percent are in Action or Maintenance. The fact that you're reading this book suggests that you've moved beyond Precontemplation regarding exercise and your mental health. If you haven't been exercising, maybe you're curious about the psychological benefits. If you're already exercising, you may be reading in order to obtain further information or support for an activity that has significance to you.

Each stage has value and purpose, and in order to really change it's important that you not rush through them. One of the biggest mistakes in beginning exercise is to spend too little time in Contemplation and Preparation. If you leap into Action but then relapse, you may feel confirmed in your belief that you are a failure and that you're just *never* going to exercise regularly. Similarly, if you're helping someone begin an exercise program and encourage a Contemplator to Action too vigorously, that person may become more resistant and retreat to Precontemplation.

A psychologist colleague of mine, Maria, is familiar with this model of change. She found a unique way around the challenge of exercise:

◼ *Maria's Story*

Exercise was such a stumbling block for Maria that she wrote her doctoral dissertation on the subject. It took over two years to make a long-lasting and significant change in her eating and exercise habits. She stayed in the Contemplation stage for much of that time.

Let's look at each of these stages in more detail and talk about some of the things you can do to get yourself ready for the next stage.

Precontemplation

People tend to be in Precontemplation for a number of reasons. You may be uninformed about the long-term effects of your behavior. You may feel unhappy and defeated, deciding that the best way to deal with your frustration is just not to think about this behavior. You may feel defensive about changing. Perhaps when you think about exercise, you immediately remember how much you hated P.E. in high school.

EXERCISE: WHAT STAGE ARE YOU AT?

In terms of exercise or sport behavior, what stage are you at right now? Here's a quick way to find out. Circle the statement that most clearly reflects your current behavior.

Precontemplation: "I currently do not exercise, and I do not intend to start exercising in the next six months."

Contemplation: "I currently do not exercise, but I'm thinking about starting to exercise in the next six months."

Preparation: "I currently exercise some, but not regularly."

Action: "I currently exercise regularly, but I have only begun doing so within the last six months."

Maintenance: "I currently exercise regularly and have done so for longer than six months."

You may have vivid memories of a particular time when you were clumsy and felt humiliated. You may leap to the conclusion that if you were to exercise now you would have the same experience. Or perhaps you tried exercise a few years ago, but what you tried didn't last more than a few weeks. Besides which, it hurt. Even though there are over fifty concrete benefits from sixty minutes of exercise, Precontemplators tend to narrow their perspective and can only list five or six.

If somebody you know is in Precontemplation, probably the most important ways that you can help them move on to Contemplation is to provide them with some information and a lot of support and optimism from your own experience. Don't be surprised if they aren't immediately enthusiastic. Don't worry if they are filled with lots of "yes, but"s. This may be a time when they talk about what hasn't worked before or how badly they've felt in other exercise situations. Yet the fact that they are even willing to read, listen, watch something on TV, or surf the Net on the subject suggests that they might be moving toward the next stage. When I spoke with Carrie, she seemed an ideal candidate for the multiple benefits of exercise.

◼ Carrie's Story

Carrie was forty and had come to see me because she was depressed and overweight. She said she wanted to change. Although she had a history of severe and chronic physical illness, she was now in adequate physical condition and was being carefully monitored by her physician. He had been encouraging exercise for a few years, and Carrie knew that she *should* exercise. Occasionally she went for a walk. Given her life situation and her health risks, walking seemed the most likely form of exercise for her. Over a number of weeks, Carrie and I talked about various environmental issues and constraints involving time of day, frequency, and duration. Each time we spoke, Carrie would appear involved and responsive, but in fact, she never followed through. Over time, she and I recognized that she had a pattern or style of sweetly not complying with other people's expectations of her. This passive resistant style in regard to exercise initiation reflected a more general stance that kept her dependent on others and hesitant about "ownership" of herself. We needed to have more extensive discussions about this style before there would be any movement toward exercise. The issue of exercise and more broadly, self-care, could then become a measuring ground for change.

Contemplation

Contemplation is a fascinating stage. You may stay in Contemplation for a long time or return to it from Preparation or Action. (Yes—unfortunately, but realistically, this model doesn't go in one direction only!) The Contemplation stage is the highpoint of ambivalence. It's the time when you are weighing options, when you're thinking: "On the one hand . . . ; but on the other . . ." This is a really important time to assess the benefits and costs of exercising (see "How Ready Are You," below). You can assess both the pros and cons of exercising. It is helpful to look at the positive *and* negative consequences to and reactions of yourself and others. Sometimes understanding the negative consequences can help you address them so that you can move to the next stage. If you develop a sense of self-efficacy for exercise (that is, a belief that you are going to be successful in this process), you will be able to move into Preparation more easily and effectively. For example, Joan, a few years older than Carrie, was also dependent and depressed.

■ Joan's Story

Joan was rapidly sinking into a deeper and deeper emotional hole at the time when she truly began contemplating exercise. She recognized that inactivity increased her depression and her sense of helplessness. She talked with a few friends, with her husband, and with her kids as she considered undertaking this change of activity and self-view. She recalled her sense of well-being and the pleasure she had experienced when she had exercised for a few months. We discussed the anticipated impact (positive and negative) her exercising might have not only on herself but also her family. She developed an increased sense that this time, with her thoughtful planning, she would be able to create an exercise pattern that she might be able to sustain.

Preparation

Making a commitment to change is the hallmark of the Preparation stage, and with that can come considerable anxiety, self-doubt—and more ambivalence. Increasing the number of pros versus cons on your cost-benefit analysis can be helpful. When you double the list of pros, you'll be ready for a stage change (Prochaska 1996).

This is the time when you try out new behaviors and see what you learn from this experience. You whittle away the negatives and increase the positives. Like Contemplation, you may stay in the Preparation stage for a long time. Another client of mine, Sara, prepared to exercise differently.

▣ Sara's Story

Having tried a number of commercial weight-loss programs, Sara entered therapy feeling discouraged about herself, her life, and her parenting skills. She was also still reeling from the effects of long-term abuse in a marriage that had finally ended three years ago.

At one point during her marriage, Sara had gone jogging on a daily basis. Now, however, she felt uncomfortable about being outside alone for any length of time: she feared that her ex-husband might stalk her. Instead of focusing on weight, self-image, and exercise, therapy centered initially on finding genuine ways she could experience power with regard to basic life issues—at work and in her continuing concerns about custody of her children.

As she began to feel competent in work and parenting, Sara was willing once again to tackle the question of her body image. She tried out various extreme diets before settling into a nondeprivation method of eating control. Although she was aware that exercise would assist in weight loss, in the past she had used exercise to "cheat" on diets: she would exercise to "balance" overeating. She decided to postpone regular exercise until she felt committed to the weight-loss program she'd designed for herself.

Sara rewarded her commitment to her eating plan by buying a treadmill. She thought through the logistics carefully: when she would use the treadmill, where she should place it so that she would actually use it, and how she would act gradually in building up her use. A weekly graph of weight loss and exercise helped her see change over the long term and reinforced her sense of competence.

Action

Action is the "on" stage, the time at which actual behavioral change has taken place with some consistency. It's also the stage with the highest risk of relapse. To avoid slipping back, pay attention to both the tangible and abstract obstacles in your way and address these difficulties in a systematic way. Observe the ways in which your environment supports the change you've made. For example, Ron, a twenty-six-year-old lifeguard at the pool where I swim began running again during Chinese New Year.

▣ Ron's Story

Ron had made a New Year's resolution to himself to start running more regularly, but he got a cold after two days and stopped. Chinese New Year, a few weeks later, became the occasion to mark a new start.

Ron had always thought of himself as an evening runner, even though he never really consistently ran in the evenings. He realized that because of his schedule, he had a free block of time midmorning. Now he's using this time three days a week to run forty-five minutes at a time. He's found a running route that he likes down along the lake and he's feeling enthusiastic. He smiles broadly as he says, "It's great. I have more energy. I'm sleeping better. Back when I was running at night, I slept, but it was kind of a restless sleep. Now it's deep." And because he and I have been chatting about the subject of exercise for months, he says that my voice is in his head with each footfall. "It's a lifestyle change; it's a lifestyle change," is his current mantra.

At the Action stage, it is especially helpful to keep behavioral records of your activity. Your Exercise Log (see chapter 4) will be a central aspect of this stage.

Maintenance

Maintenance involves processes similar to the Action stage. It's important to focus on those methods that reinforce your behavior change. Two factors are central to maintaining changed behavior of any kind over time: sustained, long-term effort and revision of your lifestyle. You come to recognize: "I really *am* capable of doing this behavior over a long period of time." Your lifestyle undergoes some changes—and it's important to notice what these are. Are you getting up earlier? Have you found the most convenient gym? What is it that you're doing less of? (There are still only twenty-four hours in a day—despite our best efforts to find additional minutes or milliseconds!) Although these may be small and subtle changes, they are the ones necessary to guarantee that you're going to maintain what you have put into action.

Beginning to exercise and continuing to exercise are two connected actions—but they're not the same. Let's start at the beginning. We'll address the issue of maintenance in chapter 9.

How Ready Are You?

A useful way to figure out your readiness is to look at the pros and cons of exercising. This "cost-benefit analysis" involves both you and those around you. Fill out this analysis as completely as possible. If the negatives outweigh the positives, you probably aren't quite ready to make the exercise change yet. It will be important to focus on:

1. Increasing the number of benefits;

2. Eliminating or reducing the negatives;

3. Recognizing the relative value of certain items. Some reasons are more important than others. You can "weigh" them differently.

(And remember: the very process of completing this chart helps you understand your motivation and brings you closer to making changes.)

EXERCISE: YOUR EXERCISE READINESS

How ready are you to exercise? If you are not currently exercising, this is a moment, as the Alcoholics Anonymous phrase goes, to take a "fearless inventory" of yourself. As you were reading about the stages of change, perhaps you noticed some resonating thoughts or feelings in yourself. To make this more specific for you, what is your "Yes" or "No" answer to the following questions? Do you:

Y   N   1. Think exercise is irrelevant and you're not considering exercise?

Y   N   2. Think that you probably should exercise?

Y   N   3. Have some interest in exercising?

Y   N   4. Try to do some form of exercise, such as taking a fifteen minute walk, at least occasionally?

Y   N   5. Exercise, predictably, at least thirty minutes at least three times a week?

- If you responded "Yes" to number 1, it is impressive that you've read this far in this book! Although you're saying that you are in the Precontemplation stage of change, your *behavior* suggests that you are in Contemplation.

- If you answered "Yes" to number 2, you've moved into Contemplation. Getting information, such as you are doing with this book, will directly assist you in making additional changes.

- If your reply to number 3 was "Yes," you're most likely on the way to Preparation, and again, getting more information and applying it to yourself and your circumstance will help you progress.

- If you're actually exercising some of the time ("Yes" to number 4), you are well into Preparation.

- And if you're exercising on a predictable and regular basis ("Yes" to number 5), you are in the Action (if less than six months) or Maintenance (if more than six months) stage. You are probably reading *Move Your Body, Tone Your Mind* to understand more about the mental benefits that you're getting or could get from exercise, or perhaps you are looking for a new way to support and reinforce your habit.

- -

EXERCISE: COST-BENEFIT ANALYSIS

Date _____

Issue: If I _____ (for example: If I begin exercising)

The mental benefits will be: The mental costs will be:

I will receive support from*:   I will be challenged by*:

(*Hint: Supports and challenges can be people or circumstances.)

- -

I think the following poem is a great illustration of change as a process rather than a static event. To me, the author's fourth and fifth sections each provide a possible ending. Sometimes we figure out ways around problems. Sometimes we direct our actions elsewhere. You can use the images in the poem to remind you of your particular holes, streets, and solutions.

Autobiography in Five Short Chapters
by Portia Nelson (1977)

1) I walk down the street.
 There is a deep hole in the sidewalk
 I fall in.
 I am lost . . . I am hopeless.
  It isn't my fault.
 It takes forever to find a way out.

2) I walk down the same street.
 There is a deep hole in the sidewalk.
 I pretend I don't see it.
 I fall in again.
 I can't believe I am in the same place.
  But it isn't my fault.
 It still takes a long time to get out.

3) I walk down the same street.
 There is a deep hole in the sidewalk.
 I see it is there.
 I still fall in . . . it's a habit.
 My eyes are open
 I know where I am.
 It is my fault.
 I get out immediately.

4) I walk down the same street.
 There is a deep hole in the sidewalk.
 I walk around it.

5) I walk down another street.

We're now ready to explore the mental aspects of beginning to exercise. We'll look at some of the internal factors that influence people's decisions, like motivation, and some of the external aspects, such as circumstances and situations. Reviewing your current behavior, your history, and your goals will be important at each step of the way.

CHAPTER 4

DESIGNING YOUR EXERCISE PLAN

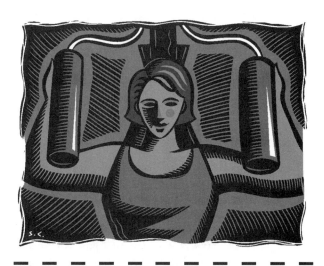

Now that we've discussed the process of change, let's focus on designing an exercise plan for you. This is a time of exploration, an opportunity to understand how your past affects your current perspective, the ways that your present life impacts your intentions, and how your goals can shape your current exercise life.

A mysterious painting by Paul Gauguin at Boston's Museum of Fine Arts asks fundamental questions of us all. Its title is: "Where Have We Come From? What Are We? Where Are We Going?" That's what we'll explore in this chapter

After defining some exercise terms, we'll examine the basic considerations for beginning and continuing an exercise program. We'll weave in physiology and psychology as we review your exercise history and current status, the type and dimensions (frequency, intensity, and duration) of exercise, and significant social and environmental factors. We'll map out your initial exercise goals. Reviewing these issues in a systematic way will give you the opportunity to design your exercise plan—and then modify it as you gain more information.

The Past Is—and Isn't—Prologue: Your Exercise History, Values, and Beliefs

Understanding your own exercise history can give you important information about yourself and your relationship with exercise. Although your past behavior, thoughts, and wishes don't determine what you will do, increased awareness of patterns and influences can give you information and guidance on directions that are likely to work for you. To understand more about yourself, you will want to do some reflecting, both in this workbook and in your journal. Many of the suggested assignments here are ones that are useful to return to and even repeat as you understand and learn more about yourself.

Your Exercise History, Beliefs, and Patterns

A history of activity tends to predict the likelihood of future activity. Thus, if you've exercised in the past, you're more likely to exercise in the future. At the same time, it's important to be aware that that same history can get in your way: You may remember past glories and either think that you should be who you once were or feel really upset that your body doesn't function exactly as it did in the past. If you are a former jock, you may start out by competing not against your age-mates but against your image of who you were twenty years ago. Inevitably, if you are out of shape as well as older, your current self will "lose." Of course, it is important to recognize and build on old skills, yet at the same time be aware of the ways in which your body is now different.

■ Beth's Story

Like many girls, in her youth and teen age years Beth loved everything about horses. She rode horses, took riding lessons, and participated in horse shows. When she wasn't riding, she read all the novels that she could find about taming wild horses. As she grew into adulthood, her life and interests shifted away from horses. A few years ago, her sister-in-law invited Beth to ride, and she eagerly responded to the opportunity. Beth's body settled into the saddle and her hands knew just how to handle the reins. Expecting to be stiff and sore after riding for a few hours, Beth was surprised that her body adjusted so easily. She was intrigued to discover that as she continued to ride over the next weeks and months, her body remembered more and more how to sit and how to work the horse.

JOURNAL TASK: THE IMPACT OF MY EXERCISE HISTORY AND EXERCISE BELIEFS

In your journal, write about the history of your beliefs about you and exercise. What impact have these beliefs had on your behavior, both in the past and right now? As a kid, were you overweight, slow, last picked? Or were you graceful and effortless in your actions but now feel dull and plodding? You can write freely on this topic, or you can start with some sentence stems, such as:

When I was eight, I was physically _____

As a teenager, I thought that my future in sports would be _____

I always thought that girls (boys) (men) (women) _____

My parents _____

My parents thought that I _____

I see my past beliefs reflected today through these current beliefs or actions: _____

_____

_____

Understanding your exercise history and your beliefs about yourself and exercise are critical components in developing patterns of exercise with which you will want to become involved. What types of exercise have you enjoyed in the past? What have you wanted to do but haven't tried? What kind of activity has meaning to you (Wankel 1993)? What types of exercise take into account some aspects of your personality? For instance, do you enjoy risk-taking or feel more comfortable with predictability? Do you want to exercise with other people or have some time to yourself? Or do you like exercise that can allow either option? What kind of financial flexibility do you have, and how much money do you want to commit to exercise? And how likely do you think it is that you will actually begin and continue exercising at this time?

- -

EXERCISE: YOUR EXERCISE PATTERNS

Remember: There are no right or wrong answers in this book. Your openness to yourself is critical to your learning. Try to use this openness as you complete this exercise.

1. Have you exercised regularly in the past? If so, when, and what did you do?

_____

_____

_____

2. What have you enjoyed? _____

3. What aspects were particularly relevant? Circle the relevant variables (and it doesn't have to be either/or—it can be both):

　　Alone vs. with others

　　Individual vs. team sport

　　Self-directed vs. program participant with instructor

　　Ease of activity vs. skill development

　　Predictability vs. thrill or variability

　　Self-focused vs. competitive

4. Are there forms of exercise or exercise programs that you have wished to participate in or thought about learning?

_____

_____

_____

5. What has been problematic? Why did you stop? How would that form of exercise/activity be difficult to engage in now?

_____

_____

- -

Now that you understand more about your past, here are some additional interesting ways to explore the relationship between you and exercise. Do you remember those classes in high school where you could earn extra points by doing additional assignments? Well, the ideas that follow are sort of like that: they aren't *necessary* to this process, but they might give you a real leg up. They are playful ways that you can learn more about your different internal "voices."

JOURNAL TASK: MY EXERCISE STORY

1. **Internal Dialogues and Letters:** Internal Dialogues are based on the assumption that we each have a variety of perspectives within ourselves, and that we can understand more about those different perspectives if they become manifest (for instance, through writing). The basic plan is to think of yourself as a scribe, listening in intently to "conversation" going on inside of you on a particular topic. As scribe, you also become the screenwriter, writing down what each "part" of you has to say.

   There are an endless number of internal dialogues you can create. Here are some of them. You could write a dialogue between the following "characters."

   - Yourself at different ages in relation to exercise.
   - Yourself and "Exercise" (or yourself and "Sports"—and by the way, what's your experience of the difference, for you?). Personify Exercise as if it had human characteristics and could hold a conversation with you.
   - Yourself and a person significant in your exercise history.
   - A variation on the dialogue is to take the position of one of these "voices." Write a letter to the other.

2. **Steppingstones** (from Progoff 1975). Regarding exercise, what have been the significant points, or "steppingstones," in the stream of your life? List about eight to ten of these and then write a paragraph about that time in your life. (Hint: You can also project into the future.) Use metaphors and similies liberally. For instance, you can describe each steppingstone by beginning: "It was a time in my life that was like _____" (a dank bog; a fresh breeze; a roller coaster).

Understanding Your History

Having completed these various reflections on your history, how do they carry forward to the present and future? Are there beliefs that you have about yourself and exercise that limit your range of possible activities and options? And on the other hand, have you rediscovered some strengths and a sense of joy in your "body-self" that you'd forgotten existed? What have you recalled or understood?

- -

EXERCISE: I'VE LEARNED THAT . . .

Write out statements describing what you have learned or relearned about yourself and exercise. If a statement has the potential to limit you, write out an alternative perspective about yourself and exercise.

I've Learned That . . .   *Alternatively:*

EXAMPLE:

"I've relearned that I avoid taking   "I can exercise in ways that don't
lessons because I think that I should   involve lessons." Or "I can let myself
already know how to do new moves,   learn—I pick up new moves really fast."
even before I've been taught."

"When I was lifting weights, I felt
emotionally strong."

_____   _____

_____   _____

_____   _____

_____   _____

_____   _____

- -

Type of Exercise

If you're going to exercise, what kind of exercise should you do? Before figuring that out, we need to define what is meant by "exercise."

Let's Start at the Very Beginning: Defining Terms

What's the difference between exercise, movement, physical activity, and sports? *Exercise* means organized, focused physical activity that involves a certain amount of exertion. It is distinguished from *movement*, which may be random. Except where indicated, it's also distinct from organized sports in being noncompetitive. People sometimes talk about *physical activity* rather than exercise, because exercise in some people's minds is weighted down with memories and beliefs and sense of obligation. Although I'm usually using them interchangeably, there are subtle differences, especially in relation to health as compared with fitness goals. *Sport*, as compared with exercise, usually emphasizes or includes a competitive element.

How much movement is enough to "count" as exercise? Health benefits begin happening when you move rather than sit still, when you're physically more active in some fashion. If you park your car some distance from your destination and walk those extra steps, if you get up from the couch to change the dial on the TV set, you are increasing your health benefits from physical activity. And becoming healthier has an impact on your mental health: you are behaving proactively to take care of yourself, you are reducing some health risks, and this form of activity can serve the function of mental distraction. Planned, structured exercise that involves the development of *fitness* strengthens muscles, provides greater flexibility, and has more profound effects on your heart and lungs. It may have more profound long-term mental effects as well.

Exercise is sometimes categorized as either aerobic or anaerobic. *Aerobic* exercise refers to activities that increase your heart rate and thus require you to use oxygen continuously over a period of time. Because of the demand placed on your body through aerobic activity, you strengthen the functioning of your heart, lungs, and blood vessels. Standard aerobic activities include walking, running, cycling, swimming, and so on. *Anaerobic* activity involves intense, short bursts of effort. This type of exercise, such as strength or weight training, sprinting, or calisthenics, builds strength through demand on your muscles more than your heart or lungs.

Some kinds of exercise emphasize endurance, while others help you become stronger, and still others increase your balance or flexibility. Your choice of exercise may be determined in part by which of these is psychologically as well as physiologically important to you. *Cardiovascular* or *cardiopulmonary* fitness (the strength of your heart and lungs) is critically important to your overall health. However, various research studies suggest that people can experience psychological improvement even if cardiovascular changes don't occur.

What's Your Definition?

An important aspect of choosing the kind of exercise that you want to try relates to what you think about different forms of exercise. If you're a woman, you may think: "Weight lifting is only for guys. I don't want to get *too* muscled." (This belief is a signal for you to get more information on the benefits and effects of weight lifting. It's also a hint that it's time to begin addressing your stereotypes about bodies.) Or you may say to yourself: "I'm too uncoordinated to play golf." (You may want to check out your general assumptions about yourself and your coordination.) You may think that certain activity is exercise but other activity isn't really. For instance, if you used to jog, you may think of walking as just a means of getting from one location to another. (This is the time to assess your current fitness level instead of resting ineffectively on old and now irrelevant laurels.)

- -

EXERCISE: YOUR BELIEFS ABOUT EXERCISE

My definition of exercise is:

_____

_____

_____

_____

_____

_____

- -

One answer may be supplied by your history, as we've discussed: what you've done, what you've liked, what you have wanted to do. Another may relate to the particular mental effect you're looking for. I say "may" because some of this is speculative. Although some research suggests that specific activities affect particular moods or thoughts, your own preference probably is the most important influence. A depressed and injured client, Roland, made this fact vividly real for me:

■ Roland's Story

It was not until well into treatment that Roland revealed that he had been physically active all along. On instruction of his physical therapist, Roland had used an exercise bicycle twice a day for the past number of months. The bicycle had, no doubt, been effective in preventing the loss of muscle tone and maintaining some physical flexibility. But it apparently had had no effect on his state of mind. It was walking that he was interested in doing and, ultimately, walking that seemed to have a direct effect on his mood.

What Are Your Exercise Options?

There are a huge number of exercise possibilities available to you. You can stick with one or mix and match. You may be looking for maximum physical benefit, lowest cost, easiest, most beloved, most calories burned, and so on. The types of exercise listed here are intended to help inspire you to find some form(s) of exercise that will work for you. Feel free to add to the list.

Aerobic dance	Rock climbing (indoor or outdoor)
Basketball	Rowing
Bowling	Skating (ice, hockey, in-line, or roller)
Canoeing	Skiing (cross-country or downhill)
Cycling (road or stationary)	Soccer
Frisbee	Softball
Golf	Strength or weight training
Hiking	Swimming
Jogging or running	Tennis
Kayaking	Walking
Martial arts	Yoga
Racquetball	

The Primary Mental Elements of Exercise

From a mental perspective, is all exercise created equal? Probably not. We can make some good guesses about the dimensions of exercise that are important in determining mental benefits. In general, certain types of exercise seem to be especially likely to improve your mood. Bonnie Berger, an exercise and sport psychology researcher at Bowling Green State University, has spent a number of years exploring the relationship between exercise and mood. She and her colleagues have found that there are some common elements. Let's review them in detail.

Getting the Most Out of Getting Moving

Optimal mental benefits from exercise are likely if:

- the activity is pleasing and enjoyable,

- the *mode* is aerobic or involves rhythmical abdominal breathing, and the *activity* is predictable or spatially certain, with an absence of interpersonal competition,

- the exercise is regularly included in your weekly schedule, of moderate intensity, and lasts at least twenty to thirty minutes. (Berger and Motl 2001)

Enjoyment is a key element in your exercise for a number of reasons: If activity is enjoyable, you are more likely to continue to do it—certainly a necessary component for experiencing the benefits of any program. And if it is enjoyable, it will add to the sense of psychological benefit that you receive. Think of the difference between the admonition "No pain, no gain" compared with "Exercise that is fun will get done!"

Rhythmic abdominal or diaphragmatic breathing, which occurs naturally when you exercise vigorously over a period of time, increases a sense of subjective well-being in and of itself. For some people, the exercise-associated changes in breathing pattern, even more than the aerobic aspect, may create the psychological benefit.

Closed environments and spatially certain activities include exercise such as walking, running, and swimming. These forms of exercise allow you to preplan your movements and predict your pattern of energy expenditure. Because they are rhythmical and repetitive, they support the potential for tuning out your environment and tuning inward instead. People often speak of the opportunity for contemplation, reflection, and creativity (see chapter 8) that such activity can allow.

Perhaps because it is so simple and common, walking might be considered the "aspirin" of exercise. When exercise is recommended, walking is probably the safest and most frequently proposed. Walking is generally the exercise of choice among physicians when they encourage their patients to exercise. It's also the favored activity for weight-loss support groups, such as Weight Watchers and medically managed weight-loss programs. Fitness walking has increased by about a third over the past decade (*The Walking Magazine* 2001). Yet few research studies have examined the effectiveness of walking on mental health. What this means is that, while walking certainly won't hurt, how much it helps appears to be an individual matter. Throughout this book, you will read about various clients of mine who have found walking to be of considerable mental benefit.

Change It Up or Keep It the Same

How much predictability or variety do you want in your exercise? Most of the research on exercise and mood has focused on running, but a number of other forms of exercise meet Berger's classification system as well. Activities that are repetitive and do not require much attention in and of themselves allow you to "tune out and tune in." Swimming and hatha yoga, for instance, may not feel strenuous, yet they are effective in altering mood.

Some people may need to adjust to tolerating the "boredom" and routine of these forms of exercise. Yet when you regularly perform these forms of exercise, you will often find diversity in the smallest of changes. The predictability can allow for variety in ways you might not have noticed otherwise, and you may discover that what you anticipated as boring feels really refreshing.

For some, variety spices up the routine and can provide different mental as well as physical benefits. At the University of Florida, Christopher Janelle (2001) compared exercise participants instructed to use different workout patterns over an eight-week period. Those who varied their routine (though in predictable ways) enjoyed their workouts more than those who were instructed to do the same form of exercise each time. For example, my friend Sam has a set but flexible exercise pattern.

◼ *Sam's Story*

After he had been running daily for seven years, forty-five-year-old Sam noticed an occasional twinge in his right knee. Deciding to act preventively, he took up swimming again. Although the pool didn't allow him the freedom to stretch to the horizons the way that lake swimming had in the past, he was surprised to find that he enjoyed the regular count as he turned at each end. Running gave him energy; swimming brought peace. Over the next few years, he alternated running and swimming, finally settling into a weekly routine of three or four days of running and two of swimming. And his knee thanked him!

Competing

Competition is a tricky factor in physical activity. The competitive element (and/or its associated aspects; for instance, the sense of connection through team membership) can serve as a motivator. The word "competition" itself is derived from the Latin meaning "to strive with"; that is, to work at being your best in the presence of others doing likewise. Yet even if exhilarating, competition can also be experienced as stressful; it can raise a number of questions and self-doubts, tension and conflict. Competition has the potential to enhance enjoyment, but there are some caveats. Tim Gallwey, who has been studying and writing about the "inner game" of sports and other aspects of performance for more than a generation, recognizes that you can experience pleasure in competition if you can bring to that enterprise a sense of harmony between mind and body, the awareness of your body in motion, the pleasures and challenges of striving with a highly skilled opponent, and a nonjudgmental attitude toward yourself (Gallwey 1997).

- -

EXERCISE: WHAT DOES COMPETITION DO FOR—OR TO—YOU?

What has been your experience with competitive sports? What aspects of competition would you like to retain? What interferes with your mental or psychological enjoyment?

_____

_____

_____

- -

Let me share with you an example of how well competitive activities *can* work. When I asked a fifty-one-year-old colleague named Stan about his involvement in physical activity, he told me how it benefited him.

■ *Stan's Story*

Playing basketball feeds my competitive "addiction." My day in the office focuses on cooperation but my "Type A" self thrives on competitiveness. Playing basketball burns off excess irritations and keeps me in contact with young, vibrant, challenging people who make me appreciate health. It cleanses my body of the day's stresses and gives me a lift into the rest of the day's activities. It has brought with it the by-product of camaraderie that only athletes seem to share and an increased appreciation of life. I actually think of it as my art form, a way to express myself creatively (within the limits of my now diminishing skills). The number one reason I play basketball is that it's the most fun I can imagine and the best thing I share with my son.

- -

EXERCISE: BRINGING THE
MENTAL ELEMENTS HOME

Using Berger's classification system and the Exercise Options list, what forms of exercise might work best for you? An attitude of curiosity will help you discover and explore—perhaps in a way that you haven't since childhood. This attitude of curiosity can also allow you to become involved in exercise without needing to judge yourself. Consider an activity that:

- Might be pleasing and enjoyable;

- Would be aerobic or involve rhythmical abdominal breathing;

- Would be predictable or spatially certain, (probably) with an absence of interpersonal competition;

- Could be regularly included in your weekly schedule.

_____

_____

_____

_____

_____

- -

The Dose, or "FIT," of Exercise

The cardiovascular prescription of exercise three to five times per week, of moderate intensity, lasting twenty to forty minutes, has often been described as the appropriate mental "dose" as well. But truly, research hasn't yet become specific enough for me to tell you what your particular "prescription" or dose should be. The good news—it means you get to take more responsibility for your own mental and physical well-being—is that you can design the program that will work for you.

How often should you exercise? How hard should you work at it? How long should an exercise session last? Exercise trainers talk about "FIT," that is, the *frequency, intensity,* and *time* (or duration) of exercise. Particularly when you're just getting started, it's important to pay attention to each of these dimensions and not to change too many at one time.

From a practical perspective, what does this mean? At first, if you are exercising daily, you would limit the length of time and intensity. Alternatively, you might make plans to start a bit less frequently, but for slightly longer. This depends in part on physiological factors such as your current level of conditioning. From a mental or motivational perspective, what's most important is to discover what works for you—not only for one week but as something that you will be able to build upon and sustain.

Frequency

If you haven't been exercising at all, setting yourself a weekly expectation will allow you to ease into exercise. A goal of three to five days a week may work well. Shifting from exercising no days a week to seven can be a large leap. If you expect that you must exercise seven days a week, what do you say to yourself if you miss one day? If you're likely to think: "Aha! I knew it. A failure again. I can't stick with anything," you might want to reassess your expectations of yourself. On the other hand, if you exercise less frequently than three times a week, you may be leaving the door open for too many rationalizations, the lack of development of habit, inefficiency, and muscle soreness with each exercise episode. And you may not be building up the accumulated positive mental effects of exercise.

Yet some people do better if they start with an assumption that they will do *something* every single day. In this case, you will want to monitor your intensity and duration very carefully.

This is a time for personal exploration. What perspective is most supportive for you—cutting yourself some slack or giving yourself a narrow structure? In general, if you're the kind of person who tends to be hard on herself, ease up a bit on your expectations. If you're the kind of person who is a perpetual excuse-finder, tightening the reins will be useful.

Intensity

One way to monitor your exercise intensity is through "perceived effort," or what feels to you like enough. Informally, you can measure your mental effort and fatigue "temperature" on a ten-point scale. What is comfortable? For how long? What feels effortful? What level of intensity helps change your mood for how long? These interesting questions can help you assess the best level of intensity for yourself. Remember that if you are just beginning to exercise, the intensity should be fairly low. Your muscles will need time to adapt to your new level of activity.

Another measure of appropriate intensity is the "talk test," that is, your ability to maintain a conversation (if desired) while exercising. And how long does it take you to recover from a single session of exercise? If it takes longer than an hour, either the intensity or duration should be decreased.

One of the primary reasons that people stop exercising is because their initial level of effort is higher than is comfortable. This issue is particularly true of men in our society. Remind yourself that exercising is not a competition—whether against someone else or your internal beliefs about how you should exercise. As an example, my friend Dave, who's twenty-eight, presents almost a caricature of what doesn't work.

◼ Dave's Story

He has a full-time job, a new family, and is a part-time karate instructor. He wants to lose the "pregnancy weight" that he gained during his wife's pregnancy two years ago. He goes on exercise binges. Recently, he began running five miles at a time, three days a week. He loved running these long distances. He pushed himself harder and harder. But then he stopped, two weeks after he started. His muscles were sore the day after he ran, and he felt very tired. He interpreted his choice to stop running as proof that he is basically lazy.

Will he let himself run only two miles a day at a slower pace, gradually building up his endurance—with the goal of maintaining his running for more than two weeks? He shrugs and repeats, "I'm just lazy."

Is there a "dose-response" interaction between exercise and its effect on your mood? Some studies have found that more intensity is connected to a stronger positive effect. A number of other studies have not found such a connection. And some reports indicate that training at too high an intensity for too long can actually decrease your mood. In part, the dose-response relationship may relate to how conditioned your body is. After a certain amount of training, some people "habituate," or become accustomed, to a particular amount of exercise intensity. Their bodies adapt to a specific level of fitness. The initial positive psychological effect may be reduced. If that happens with you, a change in the intensity may help you again experience the physiological "kick" and/or psychological response you once felt. *Increased* exertion may augment the distraction afforded by activity. Alternatively, *decreased* intensity may offer you the opportunity to pay more attention to your body—the movement of your muscles, the evenness of your breathing, and the execution of particular moves.

Time

The duration, or length of time, that you exercise may be the first measure that you take of how exercise is affecting you. In and of itself, potentially it can be of value in helping change your self-perception. Swimming two full laps in the pool, when last week you swam only one, tells you that change is happening. Incremental increases in stamina are quantifiable, and thus are indicators of the changes you've made.

Of course, you can entirely overturn these positive effects if you set unreasonable goals for yourself and don't take into account your current level of conditioning. For example, if you've only been exercising for three weeks and think to yourself: "I should be able to run for a half hour without feeling winded," any psychological benefits you might have experienced could be undermined by this unrealistic expectation of yourself.

One of the most frequent reasons that people stop exercising is because of changes in the FIT that are too rapid—especially a too-rapid increase in duration. Standard advice to runners is to increase no more than 10 percent per week. This percentage change may seem agonizingly slow. But an exercise log, such as the one in chapter 4, will help you see that you're headed in the right direction. And making this kind of gradual change has many benefits, including increasing the likelihood of remaining injury-free. This rate of change allows your body to adapt to the additional physiological stresses. Gradual innovation may not be glamorous, but it points to the positive impact of your persistence—and thus affects your beliefs about your capacity to make these changes.

How long should you exercise, from a psychological, as compared with physiological, perspective? Recent recommendations for exercise effectiveness in terms of physiological or health benefits suggests that three ten-minute periods of exercise a day can be as effective as one thirty-minute session. For some people, short amounts of exercise may prove stress-relieving in and of themselves at the time and for a period afterwards. And if you're more likely to be able to find three ten-minute moments to be active than one thirty minute period, that in itself can be reason enough to follow this prescription. As with physiological health benefits, the generally prescribed amount to gain psychological benefits suggest twenty to forty minutes a day (Berger and Motl 2001). Some people have reported that a longer period gives further benefit. You will want to determine what works best for you, physically, psychologically, and practically.

A Final Note About FIT

In addition to its actual use as a measure of change, you can think of FIT symbolically to describe movement in the process of change itself. Just as with physical training, the process of any kind of change can be measured by what happens with the frequency, intensity, and time (or duration) of that particular issue. For example, you can tell that you are in the Preparation, rather than Contemplation, stage of change when you notice that you've been thinking more frequently, recently, about the benefits of exercise. Or you might recall with great vividness a particularly pleasurable past exercise experience. Or you might feel a sense of satisfaction about the actual experience of exercising for a bit longer. Each of these is an aspect of FIT.

FIT can also be a useful way to recognize changes in your thoughts or mood. For instance, you could use FIT to recognize that your depression is lifting, if you notice that in the past month you've been sighing less often (frequency). Possibly you haven't been feeling as "down" (intensity). Or maybe your level of energy lasts longer (time). Each of these is a dimension of FIT. This also means that if there is a day when you feel

JOURNAL TASK: MY BELIEFS ABOUT MY FITNESS FOR EXERCISE

As you embark on exercise, what are your current beliefs about your "FIT-ness" level? How frequently do you think you should exercise? What level of intensity means you're *really* exercising? How long do you think you need to exercise in order to experience some psychological effects? Date and write down your current beliefs. They may be accurate now—or they may need some revision as you understand more about your body and mind and what works for you. Review and revise (as needed) your beliefs every few months.

Date   My FITness

_____   _____

_____   _____

_____   _____

absolutely rock bottom, you can be aware that, for example, you're still able to sustain your concentration on tasks. Just as muscle development is not totally uniform and linear, so other kinds of change can occur gradually, along different dimensions.

Your Time Is the Right Time

There appears to be no specific psychobiological "best" time of day to exercise, so you should consider what works best for you. Are you a "morning" person, ready to get going first thing with energy to spare? Does your body creak and groan when you get up but feel ready to move by midday? Do you need a break in the early evening, a time to transition from work to home? Figuring out some of your own psychobiology can also aid in your planning. And remember not to make assumptions. Just because "it's always been that way" doesn't mean that your body and psyche are continuing to feel the same. Particularly as you move into your fifties and beyond, you may need to listen acutely to your body's preferences. New aches, the amount of time it takes to adapt or recover, physiological responses to heat or cold—all of these and more may need to be part of your exercise equation.

▪ Tom's Story

Tom has *always* run first thing in the morning. It traditionally has helped him focus each day. He would tease his colleague Ross, who loved running but wouldn't ever run until midafternoon. Now, in his mid-fifties, Tom has noticed some mornings when his mind is ready to run but his body just doesn't seem to want to get in gear until he's been awake for a few hours. Tom has begun thinking about how and whether to modify his daily run.

Sociocultural Variables

If you're considering exercise, gender counts. We are affected both by the ways we were brought up as males and females in relation to exercise and what the current cultural expectations are about exercise and gender. Some women, for example, are initially uncomfortable with the (new) experience of salty sweat stinging their eyes. Some men appear constitutionally incapable of running without timing themselves, measuring themselves against an internal standard, and continually trying for a "personal best." Being aware of the way that your gender affects your connection with exercise will help you understand more about how you want to approach activity.

Exercise has been popularized as a middle class, white activity. Only recently has research begun to address exercise in relation to class or ethnicity Hall (1998). A new program in Washington, D.C., offers group fitness training within a traditional, African-American church setting, calling itself a "fitness ministry" (Lake 2001). The combination of social support, accurate information, and a safe and comfortable environment for activity all serve to sustain the motivation of the women participants. With or without research confirmation, you will want to understand your specific social and cultural content as you design your exercise program.

- -

EXERCISE: WHAT'S BEST FOR MY PARTICULAR SITUATION

The best time of day for me to exercise would be: _____

Because of my gender/ethnicity, exercise should include: _____

but would be problematic if _____

_____

In order to deal with these issues, I _____

_____

_____

- -

Social Supports

Although everyone says that social support is really helpful, when it comes down to the specifics, this is a complicated and somewhat individual issue. The right social supports are wonderful but the wrong ones can be devastating. Social supports may include your family members, friends, colleagues, or exercise buddies. Nonhuman resources can also be supportive. Books, magazines, TV shows, or videos about particular kinds of exercise give you information, role models, and opportunities for identification.

Particularly in the middle stages of change (Contemplation and Preparation), it's critically important to experience the warmth and empathy of others. Many programs emphasize the value of social interaction in developing exercise habits. Group activity can be important in terms of identifying with other group members, having a strong sense of commitment to the group, getting a sense of support from others, feeling excited about competition, and having the opportunity to participate in team activities. Regular contact with members of an exercise class, locker room connections, or genuine family support can all bolster your self-esteem or sustain flagging energy. Recent research suggests that in general, for men, active friends help sustain their exercise patterns, whereas for women, family support is more important (Wallace et al. 2000). Which is it for you?

If you experience negative reactions from others, your family members undermine your exercise plans with last minute requests, or you find yourself always comparing yourself negatively to teammates or your body to somebody else's "perfect" body, some of your enthusiasm may be stifled. It's important for you to look at where and how you're actually experiencing a sense of support.

Some people look to exercise as a time for relationship. For others, exercise may be a socially acceptable time to *dis*connect. If your life feels too filled with people and their demands, some of the stress relief you experience in exercise may relate to the opportunity to have time to yourself.

EXERCISE: SUPPORT COMES IN ALL SIZES

When I exercise, I will feel supported if _____

_____

I will feel threatened or unsupported if _____

_____

In order to cope with that lack of support, I will _____

_____

_____

Environmental Factors

Whether simply perceived or real, environmental barriers are among the most likely reasons why people don't start exercising or drop out shortly after they've started. For that reason, you should look carefully at the everyday factors that may particularly affect you. These kinds of barriers can include issues of access, such as physical location or expense. For example, my friend Jennifer checked out the availability of swimming pools near her home and her workplace before she started swimming.

■ *Jennifer's Story*

Although the pool near home wasn't as new or well-lit as the one near work, the hours it was open were a better fit for Jennifer's schedule. After she'd been using the pool for a while, she realized that the pool's lack of popularity was an advantage: the lanes and locker room were less crowded.

Another major environmental barrier for many people involves a lack of time, the logistics of squeezing yet one more thing into an overfull day. If you think of exercise as another obligation in your too-crowded life, you may resent the demand (even if it is coming from yourself!) and quit before you start. But if you pay attention to the ways exercising can increase your energy level and encourage you not to give in to lethargy, you may discover that you're using your time more effectively. This can help you move toward exercise. Ask yourself: What will I do less of in order to make space for exercise? And: How will exercise give me *more* time?

Solutions to Excusercizing

Dr. Michael Sachs, a professor in the Department of Kinesiology at Temple University, and Bruce Cohen at Evolution SportsScience have coined the term "excusercize" to describe the creative reasons people give for not exercising. When you begin to contemplate the whys and hows of exercise, do you find yourself excusercizing? I'll get you started with some of Sachs and Cohen's categories. Add in your own—and your own possible solutions.

Keeping Track

For information about yourself and exercise, it's important to keep track of what you do and how you react. Here is one format you can use.

JOURNAL TASK: MY EXERCISE LOG

Instructions: Make multiple copies of the worksheet on page 53 for your own use, or create a similar one on your computer if you'd rather record in that way. Your worksheet should be simple enough that you will complete it regularly yet detailed enough that you can extract information from it over time.

Write or use a symbol to describe the *activity*. Track the *distance* or *length of time*. Rate your *intensity* on a scale from 1 to 10. You can use an external measure such as a heart monitor or an internal measure such as your perceived effort. Rate your mood on a 1 to 10 scale, both *before* and *after* you exercise. How long does that mood change *persist*? Keep plenty of space for *thoughts, feelings,* and/or *ideas* that you have during or shortly after exercise. These thoughts may relate to you and exercise; they may be thoughts or feelings about yourself more generally; or they may be creative ideas and aha!s.

EXERCISE: EXCUSERCIZE AND SOLUTIONS

The number one reason that people give for not exercising is a lack of time—"I'm too busy," "I've got too much to do," "I gotta be somewhere ten minutes ago," "Exercise is too time consuming." Consider the solutions to this favorite form of excusersizing then write down your own favorite excuses and find potential solutions for them.

Excusercize	*Potential Solution*
Too little time	Increase time efficiency
	Address and rework priorities
	Do two things at once, like watch TV and exercise (but note whether this affects the mental benefit that you experience)
	Break up exercise into smaller chunks of time
	Walk/jog around your children's playing field during their practice/game
_____	_____
	_____
	_____
_____	_____
	_____
	_____

Exercise Log

Week of: _____

Activity	Distance and/or Duration	Intensity (1-10)	Mood Before	(1-10) After	Mood Change Persistence	Comments (Thoughts/Feelings/Ideas)
Mon.						
Tues.						
Wed.						
Thur.						
Fri.						
Sat.						
Sun.						

Matching the Exercise Plan to the Problem

You may find it helpful to design your exercise plan—type of exercise, time of day, and so on—to maximize the benefit for your particular problem. For example, if you're highly stressed at work, you might want to focus on an exercise program that helps reduce your resting heart rate and blood pressure. You may benefit by taking some time out to exercise. Specific suggestions matched to the issues that you may be dealing with are made in the next part of this book.

Another possibility is to use the same form of exercise for different purposes. Consider Alice's strategy.

◼ *Alice's Story*

Alice began using a stationary bicycle as part of our treatment plan to help her manage depression, anxiety, and post-traumatic stress disorder. Daily low-level cycling for twenty minutes had little effect. She increased the frequency to three times a day (and thus, the duration as well) and varied the intensity. In the morning, she would ride the bicycle for fifteen minutes to become more alert and control panic. She used this time also to visualize methods for coping with the day. In the afternoon, she pedaled at high intensity for fifteen minutes to alleviate the stresses of work and as an alternative to binge eating. In the evening, slow and comfortable, she rode for varying lengths of time as she reworked trauma issues.

Having sorted through the various aspects of your exercise program, you're now in position to think forward and to set goals for yourself.

Your Exercise Goals

One of the most important aspects of getting started is to have a plan in mind—at least an initial sense of what you want to accomplish. Setting goals gives you a framework and serves to reinforce the changes you make. Goal setting will work best if you write down your goals, have a regular method for keeping track of how and what you are doing, and regularly review and revise your goals.

Your journal will be an important ally in this process. Make sure to make it work for you. Remember that the journal tasks I'm suggesting can always be modified to suit your purposes.

The very process of observing your own behavior (self-monitoring) helps you remember to focus on that behavior, gives you accurate feedback so that you won't distort the information in your memory, provides information for review and revision of your plans, and helps you feel in control of your own behavior and plans. As with any reinforcement, specific *positive* observation and recording will serve you well. We all like to be told we're doing a good job—even when we're the ones saying that to ourselves! And positive feedback helps us understand what to do. (Saying "Don't do such and such" doesn't really give us any direction. While it may tell us what's wrong, it certainly doesn't indicate what's right.)

Setting SMART Goals

How do you go about setting goals? By being SMART. Your goals will be most effective if they are **S**pecific, **M**easurable, **A**ction-oriented, **R**ealistic, and **T**imed. What does that look like? Let's take Edward as an example.

■ Edward's Story

A thirty-eight-year-old computer programmer, Edward had been in an emotional slump. He said that he'd like to feel better about himself. But what exactly did that mean? I asked him how he would know if he felt better about himself. "I'd wake up looking forward to the day instead of dreading it. I'd hang out with the guys at lunch the way I used to instead of sitting holed up in my cubicle. I'd get back to the weekly biking group."

We started with an action that Edward could take immediately: getting involved in the biking group again. He knew where and when it met. He decided to call one of his friends who was a "regular," and tell him that he was coming that week. This public announcement would help increase the likelihood that he would follow through on his commitment.

Goal Difficulty

How high should you set the bar? How difficult should your goals be? Some of this depends on your particular personality and preferences, of course. You can review other times in your life when you've wanted to achieve something in particular. What level of difficulty got you motivated and kept you motivated? In general, goals that are somewhat difficult but attainable seem to help most people change, most of the time. But if you're trying something new or learning a difficult task, it helps to set easier goals. Shifting from the inertia of *not* being active takes energy, and the risk-taking involved in learning something new also takes energy. By being kind to yourself and giving yourself a break, you will feel more supported. On the other hand, if what you're planning to do is either very simple for you right now or familiar, then setting higher expectations for yourself will be more motivating.

■ Walter's Story

Walter had been an avid rower in college. Now forty and feeling depressed, he knew that he couldn't leap back into the full regimen of rowing, weights, and running that had sustained him as an undergraduate. He joined a fitness facility with rowing equipment. He would start with the regular rhythm of the machine, finding out how long he could sustain his stroke before setting specific time goals for himself.

Multiple Goals

Any one goal should be SMART. But what if you have only one goal for yourself and don't meet it? To avoid hitting this wall, it's a good idea to set three different goals for yourself. That way, you can learn more about yourself and exercise, finding out what changes easily and what will take different effort or a more careful appraisal of your current life circumstances.

You can also set different levels with regard to any one goal: what you expect and could live with; what you'd feel really good about; and what would be really fantastic. In the process of developing this range of goals, you may discover that in fact the "really fantastic" goal was the only one you were allowing yourself. You would be setting yourself up for major disappointment if it were that goal or nothing.

▣ Andrea's Story

At twenty-seven, Andrea had been walking regularly for six months. Whether because of winter or the recent end of a relationship, she was also aware that she was feeling increasingly moody. She was snapping at her best friend Margi, was frequently near tears, tired, and didn't have much appetite. She decided to begin running to see if it would not only improve her physical condition but help her mood as well.

Andrea set and wrote down goals for herself three months from the day she began running. She wrote:

1. I will run three days a week for a half hour at a time.

2. I will enjoy spending time with Margi.

3. I will feel energetic and have an appetite again.

Andrea also recognized that these goals might be somewhat idealistic, and so she modified each to some degree. For example, with regard to running, she wrote:

1. Just right: I will run four days a week—and maybe compete in a road race.

2. Good enough: I'll run three days a week, most weeks. I'll use this time to see if I notice any changes after I've run.

3. I can live with myself: I'll get out there three days a week, even if it's mostly still walking.

Goal Range

Sometimes it's useful to set an exact goal. But if you tend to be a fairly precise kind of person, it may be helpful to set a goal *range* instead. For example, you might develop a goal range of one and a half to two and a half hours of exercise per week. Or you might set a goal of walking ten to thirteen miles a week. The process of planning that range can be interesting in and of itself. It means that you will need to do some direct observation of your body's capacity rather than making arbitrary assumptions about what you should be able to do.

■ *Lauri's Story*

An introspective person who feels safest when she's dealing with numbers, Lauri at thirty-six is just beginning to move her body. She took a strength training class at the local Y and then began working out on her own. Keeping a written log of her repetitions, sets, and weights has felt very satisfying as she watches her progress and change over the weeks. She plans to stay committed to exercise—but has now begun looking at other classes offered at the Y. Rather than predict which type of exercise she'll do how often, Lauri sets an overall time range for herself:

"I'll exercise between two and four hours a week over the next two months and then determine which kind of exercise to do how often for how long."

Short- and Long-term Goals

As the SMART acronym indicates, one aspect of goal setting involves the length of time needed to accomplish your goal(s). It's useful to set both short- and long-term goals. Short-term goals provide immediate reinforcement. Long-term goals help you know where you're going. Short-term goals, set for the next week to few months, are the ones that will help you get started. Medium-term goals are those for the next three to six months. And long-term goals are those for the next year or so.

■ *Marty's Story*

Marty, at forty-three, has gone swimming as a way to handle tension for a number for years. He can predict that the next few months at work will be especially draining, and has chosen to swim more systematically. During this period of time, he's decided he'll swim four mornings a week rather than his usual two. He negotiates the necessary changes in child care (who will drop off and pick up which child where) with his wife. If this changed routine has as much impact on his tension as he expects, he will work on incorporating it into his ongoing life plans.

If you haven't been exercising up until now, recognize that your body may need a certain level of fitness before you'll experience the full mental effects of exercise. Of course everyone's different, but you may need a base level of stamina, intensity capability, or endurance before you can reliably count on exercise to give you the emotional boost that you want. Remember to give yourself at least six weeks of regular exercise before you make an evaluative judgment about whether it is effective.

Because you're reading this book, you probably have already thought a bit about setting goals related to how you feel about yourself as well as goals that concern how much or what kind of exercise you want to do. Initially, these may just be hopes ("I will feel energetic on the days that I exercise"; "I will feel less depressed for two hours after I exercise"). But it is by specifying some of these goals that you will be able to weigh the relative benefit of different kinds of exercise for you.

JOURNAL TASK: MY EXERCISE EQUATION

Instructions: This worksheet is a sample method for setting and keeping goals. Make multiple copies of this worksheet for your own use or create a similar one on your computer if you'd rather record in that way. This worksheet serves as your commitment to yourself and as your guide for action. It will be most effective if you review and revise it at regular intervals of about six weeks.

Below is an example of how part of your completed worksheet might look.

Example

Date: *March 10, 2002*

Date Scheduled for Review: *June 2, 2002*

Actual Review Date: *June 9, 2002*

Goals

1. Specify: (Short-term) or Long-term

    Current behavior (or thought or feeling): *Brisk walk around block 4 mornings a week*

    Goal behavior (or thought or feeling): *Brisk walk including cul de sac (1 mile) 4 mornings a week*

    Review commentary: *Worked the first week only; need to get up earlier if I'm going to do this consistently; therefore, need to get to bed 15 min. earlier, too*

    Revised goal: *Shorter walk 2x/week; longer walk 2x/week*

2. Specify: Short-term or (Long-term)

    Current behavior (or thought or feeling): *Feel as if I have no time to myself*

    Goal behavior (or thought or feeling): *Take time during walk to be present to nature and the neighborhood*

    Review commentary: *Too soon to tell if it's having an effect but I think I feel less put upon*

    Revised goal: *No revision needed. Keep noticing*

MY EXERCISE EQUATION

Date: _____

Date Scheduled for Review: _____

Actual Review Date: _____

Goals

1. Specify: Short-term or Long-term

    Current behavior (or thought or feeling): _____

    Goal behavior (or thought or feeling): _____

    Review commentary: _____

    Revised goal: _____

2. Specify: Short-term or Long-term

    Current behavior (or thought or feeling): _____

    Goal behavior (or thought or feeling): _____

    Review commentary: _____

    Revised goal: _____

3. Specify: Short-term or Long-term

    Current behavior (or thought or feeling): _____

    Goal behavior (or thought or feeling): _____

    Review commentary: _____

    Revised goal: _____

Contract with Myself

In order to meet these goals, I will do: _____ (activity/activities)

for: _____(amount of time/number of days a week)

(for length of time or distance): _____

(at an intensity of): _____

My reward/reinforcement will be: _____

_____   _____
                  (Signature)   (Date)

Reinforcement and Rewards

When you're changing behavior, it's very important that these changes be recognized and acknowledged in a meaningful way. This reinforcement helps you maintain the changes you are making and supports your sense of your capacity to change. There are a variety of ways that you can reinforce or reward your new exercising self. Most basically, your attention to what you're doing and the mental and physical benefits you are experiencing will be an internal reward—especially if you make a conscious effort to notice these benefits. Writing down your behavior and reactions helps make these benefits more substantial to you. Beyond merely noticing, actual commentary to yourself is tremendously reinforcing. This is one of those times when you are both subject and object to yourself. You're noticing and reflecting on what you are doing, thinking, and feeling. Your journal is a repository and a support in this process.

▣ *Rita's Story*

At thirty-nine, Rita has become entranced with running. Until she started, she had no idea that she would enjoy it so much. She's written in her journal about the different kinds of muscles she never knew were there. She's commented on her sense of stamina. She's reflected on the way she's more lighthearted in her contacts at work and more playful with her son.

Rita was sitting at a meeting one day and idly ran her hand down her leg to scratch a mosquito bite. What was this hard surface at the back of her leg? Oh! she realized, nearly giggling. That's my calf muscle. It's always been wobbly before.

That evening, Rita stared at herself solemnly in the mirror: "Woman," she said to her reflection, "you've got powerful legs. You are strong and sturdy." And she wrote in her journal about this deep sense of change within herself.

In addition to internal rewards, you can also set external rewards. These can be tangible or intangible rewards. For instance, buy yourself a treat when you reach a goal. Your treat can be anything from a copy of a new bestseller to that set of golf clubs you've been pining for. A new hairstyle or a day at the zoo may serve to mark the changes you've made.

Particularly with exercise, you may receive reinforcing comments from other people. If you tend (as most of us do) to quickly dismiss positive things that others say about you, or even that you notice about yourself, you might want to keep a "Kudos List" in your journal. You don't even have to wholeheartedly endorse the responses you put in this list. Your job is just to record. Interestingly, you'll find that this running commentary in your journal begins to take on a life of its own as you accumulate positive reactions. Your attitude toward yourself will begin to shift from deep inside.

JOURNAL TASK: MY KUDOS LIST

In your journal, set aside a page to record positive comments from other people as well as positive thoughts or feelings that you experience regarding exercise and your related thoughts, feelings, and behavior. This page can be set up as follows:

Date   *Commentator*   *Situation*   *Thought or comment*

Now that you've got the tools (the rationale and methods for exercising), it's time to look at specific applications. In part 2, we'll discuss the ways exercise has particular mental benefits with regard to anxiety, depression, self-esteem, and your thought process.

HOW TO BE THERAPEUTIC TO YOURSELF THROUGH EXERCISE

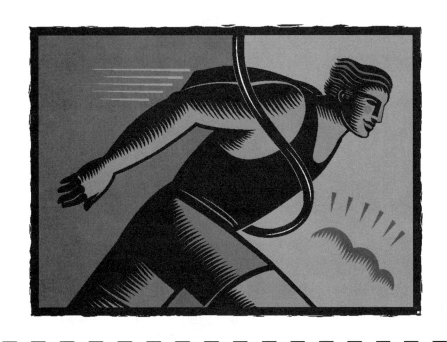

CHAPTER 5

STRESS BUSTING AND MIND CALMING

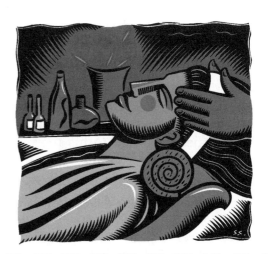

In this chapter, we'll look at the ways in which exercise is helpful for both the small and large stresses and anxieties of life. We'll start with everyday tensions, then discuss exercise in relation to clinical anxiety, and from there, to specific kinds of anxiety such as panic disorder. The first sections of this chapter describe the science (research) and practice (vignettes) of exercise in relation to stress and anxiety. The last section contains a number of recommendations concerning exercise specifically for stress and anxiety.

All Wound Up and No Place to Go

Tension and stress are parts of our daily life. We take this so much for granted that it's part of the general landscape of our existence. My friend Paul, a businessman in his mid-fifties, accepts chronic stress as a normal aspect of who he is and how he lives his life. He understands at a theoretical level that regular exercise would significantly reduce the likelihood of cardiac problems, which run in his family. He also appreciates the ways in which exercise helps him feel less stressed. Usually, however, he only does some morning stretches—when he has time. He and I spoke just before a much-anticipated holiday.

■ *Paul's Story*

Paul and his family would return every summer for three weeks to the wind-swept island they had been to many times before. He knew that the only way he could manage this much time away was by spending half the day working, responding to office crises by fax, e-mail, and phone. But he pledged to himself to walk along the beach every day for an hour or two, just being in the presence of nature.

Paul commented to me: "Walking along the ocean is a visceral, sensual experience. Sometimes I fantasize. Sometimes I work through emotions. Being in an ocean environment, I track the changes day to day along the beach and notice the effects of the wind. I just observe what's going on. My mind can do what it wants—or nothing. It gives me such a general sense of well-being. This is of course completely unlike my usual existence. It gives me such a vivid sense of vitality and renewal. The walk isn't directly related to work, yet I know the decisions I make when I come back are more complete and thoughtful. And I know I'm easier to live with."

(If this were a made-for-TV movie, Paul would have recognized on this vacation that exercise *had* to become part of his everyday functioning. Instead, I have to report that he's returned to his morning stretches and to the Contemplation stage of regular daily walking. But he certainly knows in his body and mind the mental solace of movement.)

Even in the seemingly chronic tension of our hectic lives, there are times when stress is particularly acute. When forty-eight-year-old Charlotte learned that her father had been diagnosed with a rapidly metastasizing cancer, she used walking as a way to get through her work day.

◼ *Charlotte's Story*

Charlotte felt devastated by her father's degree of illness and her own impending loss. She had been taking regular daily walks to clear her mind for a while. But throughout the last stages of her father's illness, she intentionally began using her breaks at work to walk: she walked twice around the building at mid-morning and three times at lunch. She commented, "This is what's keeping me sane." Depending on how she was feeling at that particular time, she used these "break walks" for different purposes: sometimes, what was most important was to breathe deeply and walk "mindfully." At other times, the walks were occasions for regrouping and planning.

Some of us become tense only under certain circumstances or situations. For others, anxiety is a constant companion, eating away at our enjoyment of the world. And then there are people who experience both chronic *and* acute anxiety—they are anxious most of the time and especially anxious some of the time.

◼ *Mark's Story*

Mark, a forty-seven-year-old middle manager, wanted assistance concerning serious problems with anxiety and panic. Among other things that he found effective, going to the gym on a daily basis helped to diminish his anxiety. He decided to use the gym after work, to let go of the day's stresses and feel more relaxed and energized. This gym visit also served as a transition time between work and home.

As a coach and someone who had exercised for many years (but then stopped two years before), Mark now found exercise both helpful and satisfying for him. He enjoyed "reclaiming" his body, and began seeing himself once again as powerful and capable. But he continued to worry. Because he felt insecure about his work performance, he tended to arrive at work on Mondays feeling highly anxious. He discovered that exercising before work on Mondays alleviated much of his tension.

How can you tell when you are tense? In various ways, your body tells you: your heart races, your hands become dry (or sweaty), your heartbeat picks up speed, your stomach churns, your shoulders tighten up. And your mind tells you, as well: your thoughts speed up, your focus narrows—or perhaps your thoughts become distracted. The peanut butter ends up in the refrigerator, while the jelly has been put back in the cupboard.

A tension headache, knotted stomach, or momentary sense of distraction may actually be one of the few opportunities people have to fully recognize the unity of our minds and bodies. It may not be fun—but knowing and understanding this connection can be used to your advantage.

All of us experience tension some of the time. Various terms such as arousal, tension, worry, and anxiety are used to describe this sense of agitation. Usually, arousal or tension refers to the physical ways we know we are wound up. Worry or anxiety typically refers more to the mental aspect. Of course, we aren't cut off at the neck and really experience this increase of tension throughout our entire being.

- -

EXERCISE: EXPERIENCING TENSION

Each of us tends to have certain ways that we routinely recognize tension within ourselves. Some of us notice the physical sensations connected with tension, while for others the mental sensations are most obvious. Which is it for you? In the two columns below, write down the ways that you experience tension. If you're not sure, check in with yourself the next time you're aware of being tense or worried.

Physical Sensations   *Mental Sensations*

_____   _____

_____   _____

_____   _____

- -

How tense or relaxed should you be? That depends on you, your preferences, and particular situations. Like Paul and Mark, many of us operate at a fairly high level of tension to begin with, so whatever we do that might lower that tension will be helpful. The relationship between optimal levels of performance and levels of tension is often described as an "inverted U." If you imagine an upside down or inverted U, you'll get the picture.

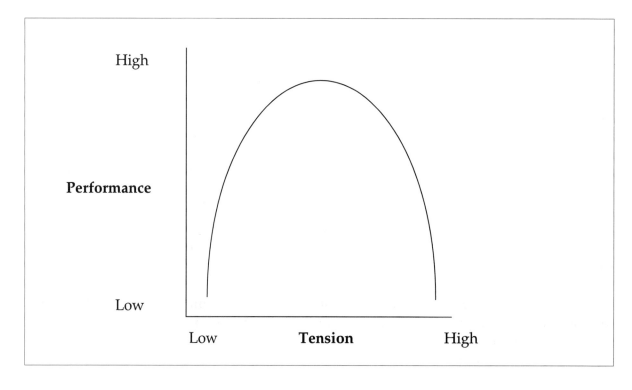

In most situations, if you don't feel any tension at all you'll be too sluggish to perform well. But at the other extreme, if you're tremendously tense, you don't enjoy yourself and your performance tends to be more prone to error. For complex tasks, up to a certain point, more tension improves performance; above that point, more tension will interfere with your performance. The challenge is to find the midrange of tension that works best for you.

EXERCISE: Your Inverted U

Think of a situation (whether chronic or acute) where you experience tension. How much is optimal for you? (Hint: It's probably less than you think!) Label the graph on the next page with the name of the situation. Write down the signs that indicate tension to you. On the inverted U on the next page, circle the range of tension that works optimally for you in this situation.

Situation where I experience tension: _____

_____

_____

Signs of tension in that situation: _____

_____

_____

_____

Optimal level of tension for me in that situation: _____

Ways that I can regulate level of tension in that situation: _____

_____

_____

_____

_____

_____

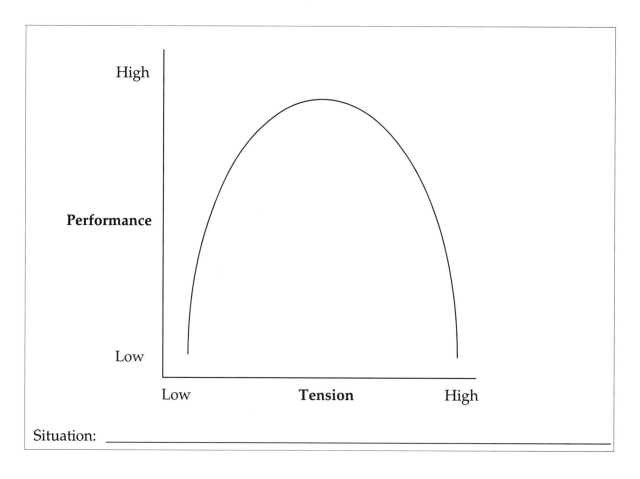

High

Performance

Low

Low   **Tension**   High

Situation: _____

What's the relationship between the inverted U and exercise? Well, exercise is one of the very best ways you can control or regulate your level of tension. Exercise has a direct impact on tension in a number of ways:

- It helps you calibrate tension;

- It helps you dissipate tension;

- It helps you to distinguish between tension and relaxation;

- It quiets and re-directs your mind.

"I'm All Stressed Out"

To be alive is to experience stressors. Hans Selye, who coined the terms "eustress" and "distress" to describe the two extremes of positive and negative stresses, suggested that finding your optimal stress level allows you to live life most fully (Selye 1975). In fact, he called stress the "spice of life." However, we usually think of "stress" as the sense of *di*stress. Distress is the difference between your beliefs about your capacities and the behavior or response actually necessary to cope with what you identify as a stressor (Berger 1994). If, for example, you are asked to complete a complicated technical report within the next few days, you may feel distressed. From this definition and example, you can see that various options exist for coping with distress: You can change your beliefs about what is stressful; you can change your beliefs about your capacities; or you can change your coping behaviors. Exercise can help you change all three. When you exercise, your perceptions and expectations about situations, other people, and yourself may change. Some of this appears to occur at a mental level, while some, we think, occurs at a physical level.

Research conducted under various conditions has repeatedly shown that people who exercise regularly recover more rapidly from stress, experience decreased stress responses, and experience fewer symptoms of physical illness in the face of negative life events.

"Stress" implies heightened levels of both physical and psychological arousal or tension. Negative moods tend to be connected with tiredness or tension. Our moods are most negative when we experience a combination of both low amounts of energy and high amounts of tension. Optimal levels of tension are the result of activities that raise energetic arousal, reduce tense arousal, or affect both energy and tension simultaneously. And exercise serves to regulate exactly these functions. "Moderate exercise has proved to be one of the most effective mood-regulating behaviors, probably because its primary mood effect is enhanced energy, but a secondary effect is reduced tension" (Thayer, Newman, and McClain 1994, p. 912). Further, since skeletal-muscular tension is a component of tense arousal, "behaviors that affect this bodily system would be important in mood regulation" (p. 912). More colloquially, you can move a muscle and change a mood.

As a society that values science and hard numbers, we tend to think that if we can measure something objectively, it's more real than subjective perception. And yet for many people who are "just" stressed in their everyday lives, the positive effects of exercise seem to be more psychological than physical. For example, one study found that, compared with a placebo group, participants in a moderate aerobic training group described themselves as less tense or depressed and more able to cope with stress—even though the *physical* measures of stress and tension hadn't decreased for either group (Steptoe, Moses, Edwards, and Mathews 1993).

Exercise and Anxiety

Anxiety and depression are the two most commonly diagnosed and treated mental illnesses. In terms of clinical definitions, generalized anxiety includes excessive, uncontrollable worry extending over a period of time about a number of situations. Typically, people who are clinically anxious experience at least three of the following: restlessness, fatigue, difficulty concentrating, irritability, muscle tension, and/or sleep disturbance. Various specific types of anxiety include panic, phobias, obsessive-compulsive disorder, and post-traumatic stress disorder.

In the U.S., approximately 7.3 percent of the adult population warrants treatment for anxiety (Raglin 1997). It's not unusual for people to be *both* depressed and anxious. For example, in various studies, up to 90 percent of patients with panic disorder were also diagnosed with major depression (Clayton 1990). And as we'll see in regard to depression, exercise can be a self-directed, inexpensive alternative or addition to other kinds of treatment.

By way of illustration, let me tell you about Gordon:

◼ *Gordon's Story*

Gordon had called for an appointment because he was feeling very anxious and was hoping for increased relaxation and self-confidence. When I met with him, he said, "I don't feel in charge of my life. I have a real problem with unknowns. I am physically tense much of the time, and I don't enjoy myself enough. I feel easily threatened by things and take criticism the wrong way. I'm just too sensitive."

Gordon had grown up with an alcoholic father who was highly critical and dissatisfied with him. For example, Gordon's father deliberately ran over his bicycle in the driveway in order to "teach his son a lesson," to remind him that he should have put his bike away.

In his late teens, Gordon was hospitalized for depression but otherwise hadn't experienced any mental or emotional problems until two years ago. Five relatives, including some he was very close to, had died within a short span of time. One day while driving, Gordon felt a severe shortness of breath, tingling in his fingers, and light-headedness. He was taken to the hospital where he was diagnosed with panic disorder. Since then, mild to moderate anxiety attacks had been a part of his daily life. He dreaded a return of the "Big One," which, despite all evidence to the contrary, he was still convinced would be a heart attack. He regularly took Xanax to diminish the anxiety.

When Gordon came to meet with me, he was dealing with some new losses in his life. He was a doting father whose only child had just left for college. Furthermore, he and his wife had recently moved to a new town and a smaller home, disrupting their previous patterns of friendship and neighborliness.

I helped Gordon understand that the various bodily sensations he described were signs that he was hyperventilating—not inhaling enough oxygen or releasing enough carbon dioxide from his body. Deep or diaphragmatic breathing would redress the oxygen-carbon dioxide imbalance, thus directly diminishing these symptoms and helping him calm down more generally.

Although he had previously exercised and played sports for years, at the time Gordon wasn't exercising at all. We discussed the ways in which being physically active would diminish his anxiety. Thinking back, Gordon remembered that exercise did help him. He enrolled in a local exercise club and began working out daily.

Gordon gradually understood that he could use his awareness of his anxiety symptoms as a cue to practice deep breathing, thus potentially decreasing the attacks or their intensity. His workouts helped stabilize his overall sense of tension and anxiety at a lower level. It took him a while, however, to get used to being less worried. He went to a jazz concert, for instance, and was startled—and then felt nervous—when he noticed that he *wasn't* uncomfortable in the small, crowded room. Gradually, he adjusted to and began enjoying his sense of increased emotional freedom. Over time he decreased his use of medication, though he continued to carry a few pills with him "just in case."

Exercise to Inhibit Panic Disorder or Agoraphobia

What happens to your body when you exercise vigorously? Your heart speeds up, your breathing becomes faster, and you become sweaty. And what happens if you're in the midst of a panic attack? Your heart races, you breathe faster, and you feel sweaty. If somebody is prone to panic attacks, it might seem like it would make sense *not* to have them go through all those symptoms again. And forty years ago, some research was interpreted to suggest that exercise might create panic attacks in people with panic disorder. Because of this early research, panic disorder patients are sometimes advised against exercise.

Fortunately, there has been considerably more research on this question, especially in the past few years. A professional article that summarizes these studies answers the question with its title: "Physical activity does not provoke panic attacks in patients with panic disorder" (O'Connor, Smith, and Morgan 2000). Both field studies and laboratory studies suggest that people with panic disorder are not likely to experience panic attacks when exercising. And, turning things around, exercise is sometimes used as a method for *assisting* people in overcoming panic attacks.

Let's look at these conclusions in detail, using some actual case examples. My client Hilda provides one illustration.

◼ *Hilda's Story*

Hilda was semiretired at age sixty-one, but enjoying life less and less. Her entire adult life had been filled with frequent agoraphobia (fears of being outside of home alone or in a crowded place) and panic attacks. Increasingly, she kept a vigilant eye on her window: were her sisters, who lived next door, at home in case she needed them? What if she didn't feel well if she was out on the road? She spent much of her time worrying and planning—anticipating disaster.

Hilda and I talked about a number of ways that she could feel less concerned and more in control of her life. We developed a list of all the methods that she could use to decrease anxiety and cope with panic. Hilda began making notes on her daily calendar of the amount of anxiety she was feeling, whether she had or hadn't had a panic attack, and what coping methods she used at various times during the day. As she became more curious about what was happening, she could begin to see patterns—and appreciate the ways that she could influence her feelings rather than be overwhelmed by them.

For many years, Hilda had enjoyed going walking at least occasionally. Now, walking became a regular, daily activity and one to which she looked forward.

Hilda and I worked together, at first frequently, and then once a month for support and checking in. Toward the end of this time, I asked her to write out her thoughts about why exercise was important to her. She started by describing her walking route in great detail, focusing on particular gardens she passed, places she had worked, her beloved church, evocative scents and their mental associations, her own long history in her neighborhood, and connections with other people. At times, friends joined her on her walk or she paused to chat. She enjoyed surveying ways that she and others had improved the community. "When I walk it's a time to be with me. It not only helps me to shape up physically, but it's a peace-of-mind time. Walking seems to help me focus. It makes me breathe deeply, and it helps to strengthen my legs, my arms, my whole body, and especially my mind. As people see me on my route and I am smiling, I wonder if they know how much this means to me. No, they probably don't know why I'm smiling—but I know and that's all that matters."

Nearly thirty years ago, an English psychiatrist tried a novel approach with patients who had long-standing panic disorder. Arnold Orwin had his patients walk rapidly or run to a designated place where their anxiety symptoms typically occurred. They arrived, of course, out of breath and with their hearts beating rapidly. As they repeated this action a number of times, they quickly learned to feel comfortable with these physical sensations rather than worry about them. For the first time in a long while, they felt a sense of accomplishment. For example, Orwin described a housebound forty-five-year-old patient who had had panic attacks for the previous thirteen years. She responded rapidly to this treatment method and Orwin concluded: "Not only was she completely free from all symptoms, but she was very confident because she felt that by her own effort she would have the ability to overcome any tendency to relapse" (1973, p. 177).

David Barlow, a psychologist who conducts research at Boston University, has developed methods for the treatment of anxiety disorders. Instead of letting clients avoid situations where they might experience anxiety, he recommends that clients be directly exposed to the situation or sensations that make them uncomfortable. They gradually learn to overcome this discomfort. In a dramatic turnaround from the belief that anxious clients shouldn't exert themselves, Barlow (1997) makes use of the physical sensations people experience when running. Aware of the physiological cues that would typically trigger a sense of panic, clients learn to redirect their thoughts and breathing when they experience these sensations while running so as not to feel alarmed. They can then transfer this thought and breath training to their everyday lives. Clients develop a sense of personal capacity and control rather than fear and avoidance. The experience of my client Sandy illustrates this transformation.

■ Sandy's Story

Sandy retired early from teaching in order to be able to spend more time playing tennis. She wasn't ever going to be a champion, but she loved the game and played as often as she could. She was a quiet, apologetic woman, always eager to please but sure that she was at fault.

As she continued playing tennis and working out, she noticed increasing problems with her breathing. She had trouble catching her breath and sometimes felt as if she were choking. She sought medical advice and saw a number of medical professionals. Various tests were conducted, but her problem defied diagnosis.

During a treadmill test designed to check Sandy's lung capacity, she began having difficulty breathing. She felt more and more worried, and finally, desperate, she screamed. The sports medicine physician stopped the test immediately. Sandy didn't develop any more symptoms, eventually calmed down, and returned to being able to breathe without difficulty.

This sports medicine physician referred Sandy to me. Although he wasn't at the time convinced that Sandy's problems were all psychological, he understood that she was a generally anxious woman and thought that talking might help.

In conversation with Sandy, it was immediately obvious to me that she was generally a very anxious, unassertive woman with extremely low self-esteem. It also seemed likely that her shortness of breath might indicate panic attacks. I explained anxiety and panic to Sandy and helped her begin to pay attention to the ways in which the exertion of exercise itself makes one short of breath. I taught her relaxation exercises, and we also talked over a few sessions about her life and various problems she had encountered along the way.

Sandy learned how to calm herself down throughout the day. She taught herself to reinterpret physical sensations as being related to physical exertion rather than impending physiological catastrophe. Over time her breathing became more predictable and functional.

The final test came the day that Sandy got back on the treadmill for another breathing capacity test. Sandy and I had spent time rehearsing how she would go about doing this test—how it would feel and what she would say to herself during it. The test was designed to stress her body to the maximum, and her physician reminded her of that. Sandy started running. The doctor and I stood by and watched, commenting to her occasionally as she ran. Forewarning her, the physician took the measure of breath capacity—and Sandy kept running. It was a strenuous task. As the clock ticked down the time, Sandy's expression became one of awe and amazement. The look of triumph on her face was wonderful to watch.

Whether you're just normally tense or stressed or have a fully-diagnosed anxiety disorder, how does this information apply to you? Let's look at some practical answers.

Body-Mind Balance

Physical activity is the primary way that we are discussing quieting the mind, yet there are other routes as well. If you're not yet familiar with them, they bear learning about. If you are already familiar with them, remembering to make use of them is often the major obstacle you'll need to overcome. Each of these methods can be used in conjunction with exercise, as you'll see. For more detail on these methods, consult a book such as *The Relaxation and Stress Reduction Workbook* (Davis, Eshelman, and McKay 2000) or a video that gives more complete instructions and variations.

Diaphragmatic Breathing

How do you breathe? Because breathing is so central to our being alive, you may not have given this question any consideration. But check it out, now.

EXERCISE: BREATHING LIKE A BABY

Instructions: Stand up and put your hands at your waist so that your middle fingers are touching. Breathe the way that you normally do. Notice the point at which those middle fingers separate and the point at which they come back together. Do your fingers part as you inhale or as you exhale? (Or do they not move at all?) Most of what I'll describe in this book doesn't have a right or wrong answer, but when it comes to breathing, there *is* a right way and a wrong way. Or at least right and wrong if you want to have your breathing work *for* rather than *against* you.

My middle fingers separated when I (circle one):   inhaled   exhaled

If you found that when you inhaled, your middle fingers separated, you are using *abdominal* or *diaphragmatic* breathing. You're bringing in enough oxygen to support your body and exhaling enough carbon dioxide to rid your body of waste products. This is the natural way that we breathe when we're born. It's the kind of breathing that occurs when we're involved in strenuous physical activity.

If, on the other hand, your middle fingers separated when you exhaled or didn't separate at all, your breathing is described as *chest* or *thoracic* breathing. You've probably been well trained to a military posture (male) or to keeping your stomach flat at all times (female). You've also trained yourself, unfortunately, to *increase* your level of anxiety—just through this shallow form of breathing.

Having diagnosed your breathing, what now? Well, if your breathing is already diaphragmatic, there are various ways that you can work with this form of breathing to decrease your level of stress or anxiety. You can focus on the breathing itself, you can develop breath patterns, such as inhaling and exhaling to a certain rhythm, or you can use the breathing as the basis for other forms of relaxation. Mostly, it's important to remember to use this form of breathing and to understand that it can directly decrease your level of tension. Often I find that people have learned diaphragmatic breathing, for example in vocal training or childbirth classes, but haven't made the transition to breathing this way in everyday life.

If you still need to learn how to do diaphragmatic breathing, here are some methods. Some people catch on really fast. Others take a while to learn. But don't be discouraged. You *used* to breathe this way—so surely you can learn again!

EXERCISE: LEARNING TO BREATHE—AGAIN

Here are some methods to help increase your awareness of your breathing and help you shift toward diaphragmatic breathing:

1. **Picture the process.** In simplified form, your lungs are like balloons, filling up and emptying out. Since your rib cage prevents you from feeling that expansion and contraction directly, you can be aware of this process by imagining that this "balloon" is located in your abdominal organs, just below your waist. Letting that "balloon" fill up and empty out is all you need to do.

2. **Start at "the end."** If you start this process by exhaling completely, you will have created a vacuum that requires filling by your inhalation.

3. **The hands know.** Put one hand on your chest and one on your abdomen. See if, just by placing your hands differently, you can keep your chest (and shoulders) still while all the work occurs in your midsection.

4. **Lie down and relax.** If you have difficulty finding this breathing pattern while standing (or sitting), lie down on your back. Again, one hand on your chest and one on your abdomen will help guide your breathing.

5. **The "book method."** Alternatively, place a book on your stomach and see if you can get it to rise and fall with your breathing.

6. **Keep it smooth.** As you begin to feel the rhythm of diaphragmatic breathing, remember to keep it smooth and even.

Diaphragmatic or deep breathing can be incorporated into any aspect of your life as a means of regulating how tense you feel. Remember the inverted U? Diaphragmatic breathing is a direct way to control your level of tension. And physical activity that incorporates diaphragmatic breathing helps you control tension.

Relaxation Methods

Both Progressive Relaxation (PR) and Autogenic Training (AT) are methods that help you relax by becoming aware of tension and relaxation in various muscle groups. PR involves a systematic sequence of actual muscle tightening and relaxation, while AT helps you focus on the sensation of relaxation, with its accompanying awareness of warmth and heaviness in those particular muscle groups. You can learn the various steps through books on relaxation or, often, sport psychology. Yoga classes typically conclude with some form of relaxation.

Meditation

Meditation has been practiced in Asia as part of everyday life for thousands of years. It has gained ground in the West over the last thirty years, popularized by the Beatles and given more practical application through Dr. Herbert Benson at Harvard. In its essence, meditation involves learning to quiet your mind, whether through focus on one particular mental object (such as a word) or gently being aware of the thoughts that drift through. Traditionally, meditation has been conducted while in a seated posture. However, it can be practiced during activity as well, as I'll describe below.

Exercise for Stress and Anxiety

The research literature and my experience in practice suggest that there is no one type of exercise that is exactly right for the reduction of stress or anxiety. The standard recommendation of aerobic exercise three times a week at moderate intensity for thirty minutes is certainly a safe plan—but your particular situation, experience of stress, and experience of stress relief through exercise may dictate otherwise.

With that forewarning in mind, let me make some suggestions. Whether your primary issue is tension or stress, whether it's anxiety, or whether it's another problem altogether but tension and anxiety are a part of the picture, I encourage you to weigh the following suggestions for yourself. Perhaps they'll ring true. Perhaps they'll spark some further ideas of your own.

Two-fers

Exercise that maximizes diaphragmatic or deep breathing has the benefit of providing tension regulation through breathing as well as the exercise itself. You get a "two fer the price of one" effect: the exercise itself is helpful and the deep breathing further serves to reduce tension. There are two quite different kinds of physical activity that emphasize diaphragmatic breathing:

1. Aerobic activities, such as running, swimming, bicycling, or skiing, require full use of your lungs, so you will automatically breathe deeply.

2. Hatha yoga typically emphasizes relaxed breathing and often includes relaxation training, a method of calming yourself. Other Eastern disciplines such as tai chi retain the element of focused breathing but may include more continuous activity. Some people feel too restless to engage in yoga and turn to the activity of tai chi as an important element in their anxiety management.

"Noncompete" Clauses

Activities that are noncompetitive are more likely to decrease tension or anxiety than those in which you're expected to perform to a certain standard. Noncompetitive activities are designed to help you remove the stressful element of judgment, whether of yourself or your opponent.

How to Avoid Chewing Your Cud

If you are "ruminative," that is, someone who tends to review and re-review your thoughts or actions, you can distract yourself from these thoughts by engaging in exercise. This is especially true for forms of exercise in which you need to pay attention to the exercise itself. Various methods for doing this are possible:

1. Use repetitive activities as a way to train yourself to redirect your thoughts to the activity itself rather than your distracting thoughts.

2. Learn a new exercise skill or involve yourself in some new moves or refinements.

3. Focus on specific elements of the activity, such as the breathing itself.

Flexible Thinking

You can control your anxious thoughts *during* exercise either through associative or dissociative strategies of thinking. If you think *associatively* while exercising, your attention is drawn to the elements of the exercise itself, whether it's your movements, your coordination, or your physiological response. When you think *dissociatively* as you exercise, your attention is directed toward other-than-just-exercise-at-this-moment thoughts.

There is no one right way to direct your thinking, but it's helpful to know that you've got a choice. For example, if you're swimming and thinking associatively, you could redirect your attention from tension or anxiety to the sensations involved in pulling your arms through water. If you run, you could focus on the depth of your breathing. Often, you can enhance associative thinking by changing the intensity of the exercise. Alternatively, dissociative methods could involve developing and repeating an affirmation in rhythm to your activity or counting the ratio of steps to breaths.

The People Factor

Sometimes we are so wrapped up in our own thinking that being with other people, especially in a planned and predictable way, can reduce stress. The company of locker room chatter can draw you out of yourself. Engagement with your team can distract and redirect your thoughts from those rattling around in your head. Yet for other people exercise may be the one moment to legitimately have time to yourself without being stressed by other people.

Mindful Exercise

Combined exercise and meditative techniques may further enhance the stress-reducing properties of exercise. You can combine some of the cognitive techniques (those that are directed toward your mind) with somatic techniques (those that are directed more toward your body). Thus, for instance, you can pair meditation with rhythmic, smooth, repetitive, noncompetitive individual activities that do not demand either complete attention or unusual alertness (Benson 1984; Green 1995).

The guru Thich Nhat Hanh describes mindful meditation as involving an awareness of your breathing and walking, so that the walking is designed for enjoyment of the present moment rather than to arrive somewhere. To walk mindfully, walk a bit slower than normal pace and coordinate your breathing with your footfalls. You might take three or four steps to one breath.

In a poetic and evocative manner, Nhat Hanh instructs and illustrates the method and meaning of mindfulness mediation:

> Each step we take will create a cool breeze, refreshing our body and mind. Every step makes a flower bloom under our feet. We can do it only if we do not think of the future or the past, if we know that life can only be found in the present moment. (Nhat Hanh 1992, p. 29)

As you walk or run, you can focus on the rhythm of your breath, saying "in" and "out" silently to yourself as you inhale and exhale, or you can count the ratio of your footfalls to your breaths. Likewise with swimming, you can focus on your breathing or use your arm motions to think "left" and "right." Feeling calm while pushing the pedals of a stationary bike, you can practice or rehearse upcoming stressful events.

Remember to Rate Yourself

The more stress you're experiencing, the more improvement you'll see through exercise. If you keep track of your subjective rating of stress before and after you exercise, you will have a direct and personal measure of the powerful impact of exercise on stress or anxiety. Use your Exercise Log to write down your level of stress on a 1 to 10 scale both before and after you exercise. Keeping track of how long that effect lasts will be another interesting and useful measure for you.

You can also keep simultaneous ratings of different aspects of tension and the effects of exercise. For instance, if you are someone who is depressed as well as tense, you could track both levels of tension *and* levels of depression before and after exercise. You might notice: "I was still just as depressed, but I felt less tense after exercising." In that case, exercise may have a direct impact on your level of tension, but you might need other types of assistance to deal with your depression. Or you might want to explore different forms of exercise.

A Potpourri of Possibilities

Because stress and stress management means so many different things to different people, exercise can have many stress-reducing features. Here are some examples:

Sometimes you need a break from what is stressing you. Exercise can act as a sort of "time-out," whether it's literally from the *thing* or task that is stressing you, or from *thinking* about the thing that is stressing you.

You can use your exercise time to focus directly but differently on the stressor, using exercise as a time to work creatively on problems or their solutions (see chapter 8).

As the information and case examples above illustrate, exercise can become a way for you to reinterpret some of the physical aspects of anxiety and panic.

CHAPTER 6

GETTING UP WHEN YOU'RE FEELING DOWN: OVERCOMING INERTIA AND CHANGING YOUR MOOD

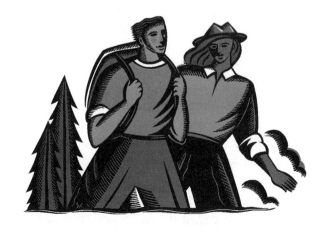

Ask someone how they feel after they exercise and, almost always, their response will be "I feel good." Exercise clearly has a direct effect on our mood—whether we're feeling a bit sad or really way down at the bottom of the pit. There's research to support this perception as well: Numerous studies of people who exercise regularly as well as athletes have shown that, compared with their mood beforehand, after exercise most people feel less depressed, less tense, less angry, less fatigued, and more energetic. Let's examine exercise in relation to depression across the wide spectrum, starting with everyday blues, moving on to grief, and then to clinical depression.

Feeling "Down"

All of us feel down some of the time—despondent, discouraged, sad—whether about a temporary or permanent loss. In a recent random telephone survey of two thousand adults in six major U.S. cities, one-fifth of those surveyed experienced some level of mood distress, whether having frequent low mood (10 percent) or meeting the criteria for clinical depression (12 percent). Signs of frequent low mood included difficulty sleeping, poor appetite, fatigue, difficulty in concentrating, and an ongoing case of "the blues" (One in five Americans 2000). Just recently, my friend Wendy called me.

▪ Wendy's Story

At thirty-two, Wendy exercises sporadically. She regularly starts running—and just as regularly, something interferes and she stops for a while. But she uses her bicycle for transportation around the city some of the time and she practices yoga, sometimes diligently—for a while. A long bike ride will leave her feeling tired and glowing, having enjoyed the air and the scenery. She feels mellow and calm after a yoga class.

Wendy called one Saturday following a recent fight with her boyfriend. Uncharacteristically, her voice was low and slow as we chatted. There was a yoga class later that afternoon, and we decided to attend. The combination of breathing, stretching, specific sustained poses, and focused concentration on something other than her relationship issues left Wendy with a sense of peacefulness and perspective about her current situation.

People use various methods to counteract negative feelings. Exercise is one of these methods, and it has powerful effects. Larry Leith, a professor of physical and health education at the University of Toronto, suggests that the primary psychological benefit of exercise is that it can help us maintain positive mental health. "Almost everyone experiences temporary, minor mood swings over the course of a day. Participation in an ongoing exercise program may serve to 'buffer' these negative feelings on a day-to-day basis, thereby resulting in lower cumulative depression" (Leith 1994, p. 32). Let me tell you about how my friend and colleague Ted has been coping with grief.

■ Ted's Story

Ted is a fifty-one-year-old professional who has been aware of his own mood changes for years. He controls mild depression through regular exercise. Without fail, he runs five to seven miles three days a week, usually starting out in the morning while it's still dark outside. Sometimes he runs with a neighbor, but often he's alone. Recognizing that he was still grieving the death of his close friend and colleague Joe, Ted told me the following story:

"I dedicated one particular run recently to my friend Joe who died last fall. I had had a really good piano lesson the day before in which a new piece I had written was well-received by my instructor, and he encouraged me to title it. I decided to call it 'Where's Joe?' On my run the next day, I allowed myself to go over a number of the pieces I've worked on over the last year and improvise in my head in a way I'm not yet able to do very successfully in everyday life. It was a wonderful, creative, poignant time. On that day and many days since, I've gone well beyond the issue of my subjective experience of being mired in loss to making my runs a healing time of remembering, grieving, and creating."

Although sadness, loss, and grief are common—and important—aspects of the human condition, clinical depression is experienced as qualitatively as well as quantitatively different. Depression both is and isn't like a more profound version of the mood shifts described above. Like the FIT acronym, part of what defines clinical depression has to do with frequency, intensity, and duration of symptoms. There also are specific symptoms that characterize depression. Among them are some combination (varying by individual and circumstance) of depressed mood or loss of interest or pleasure combined with at least four of the following: sleep disturbances, weight loss, changes in appetite, restlessness, fatigue, feelings of worthlessness or excessive guilt, impaired thinking or concentration, and recurrent thoughts of death.

Let's look at exercise in relation to these more ominous symptoms.

Exercise and Depression

Can exercise really decrease depression? My favorite illustration in response to that question comes from Kenneth Cooper, the aerobics guru who thirty-five years ago almost single-handedly helped the general public begin paying attention to the relationship between exercise and health. As recounted by sport psychologist Wes Sime (1996), Cooper told the story of a man with heart disease who was depressed:

[He] was so despondent that he wanted to die. Because his heart was weak, he thought the best way to commit suicide without embarrassing his family was to run around the block as fast as he could until he killed himself. After several futile attempts at causing a fatal heart attack in this manner, he discovered to his surprise that he began to feel better and eventually chose to live instead of to die. (p. 176)

Of all the clinical issues for which exercise has been recommended, depression has been most frequently and commonly studied (Martinsen 1990). In a meta-analysis (an analysis that statistically summarized eighty studies of exercise and depression), North, McCullagh, and Tran (1990) reached the following conclusions:

- Exercise was a beneficial antidepressant both immediately and over the long term.

- Although exercise decreased depression among all populations studied, it was most effective in decreasing depression for those most physically and/or psychologically unhealthy at the start of the exercise program.

- Although exercise significantly decreased depression across all age categories, the older people were (the ages ranged from eleven to fifty-five), the greater the decrease in depression with exercise.

- Regardless of gender, exercise was equally effective as an antidepressant.

- Walking and jogging were the most frequent forms of exercise that had been researched, but all modes of exercise examined, anaerobic as well as aerobic, were effective at least to some degree.

- The greater the length of the exercise program and the larger the total number of exercise sessions, the greater the decrease in depression with exercise.

- The most powerful antidepressant effect occurred with the combination of exercise *and* psychotherapy.

These conclusions suggest that exercise has both short-term and long-term effects; that its helpfulness in relieving depression is not specific to any one group or type of person; that the unhealthier you are, the more of a positive impact it may have; and that if you're depressed, a combination of exercise plus psychotherapy is most helpful. A client of mine illustrates this last point:

■ *Prentice's Story*

Although Prentice was only forty-two, he seemed much older than his years the first day he shuffled carefully into my office. His ten-year-old daughter had died from leukemia five years before, and since that time, Prentice had experienced severe back pain. Now he'd gotten to the point where he couldn't move with any comfort. Anticipating and afraid of additional pain, he tightened his body protectively, which tended to increase his pain in the end. He found himself involved in a vicious cycle of pain and fear. Some months earlier, with the encouragement of his orthopedist and a physical therapist, he had been able to walk a few miles a day. But his "back went out" again, and as he faced a cold and icy winter, Prentice felt emotionally and physically near paralysis.

With Prentice's permission, I spoke with his physician. The physician, who said there was no physical basis for Prentice's pain, was himself feeling discouraged about the best way to treat his patient. At this point, the physician was treating him primarily with antidepressant medication.

For several reasons, exercise seemed to me to be an essential aspect of Prentice's treatment. In the past, he had in part defined himself through athletics. Throughout his school years, he played various sports. As an adult, he was a fierce racquetball competitor. Now his pain and tightness served as a constant reminder that he was not "himself." Becoming active again would help him regain a sense of connection to his earlier self and support his development toward a feeling of wholeness. Also, if he could *see* that he was making actual progress, he might experience a sense of hope and a reason for living. On a practical level, if he had increased muscular flexibility, the risk of further injury to his back or other parts of his body would decrease. Prentice himself commented that when he was more active, he felt physically better—and more positive about himself. And finally, if Prentice were more active he might have more contact with other people (he had been becoming increasingly withdrawn).

Prentice knew that he wasn't up to playing racquetball at this point, but he remembered how much he had enjoyed the walking that he had done some months before. We discussed opportunities and options available to him, given his work schedule and fears of falling. Prentice rejoined his racquetball club, but this time he used the indoor track to walk.

Within a few sessions, Prentice was obviously moving with greater ease. Emotionally, he seemed more comfortable as well. He was much less angry, stubborn, and unpleasant (all, no doubt, aspects of the depression that had been weighing him down). He had begun walking at the club and had also started walking around his office building during the work day. He enjoyed the social atmosphere of the health club. He even began to wonder about using the club's Nautilus equipment when he was ready. Prentice described himself as already feeling and acting considerably more friendly toward coworkers.

As Prentice began to move more easily at a physical level, he also was able to make use of therapy to begin becoming less emotionally tight and closed. He started to deal with his locked up feelings about his daughter's death. With increasing emotion, he related her last moments and funeral. He brought in pictures of her and told stories about her in great detail. Each week thereafter, he would walk casually into the office, comment that he was feeling fine, report on how frequently he had walked, and then spend the remaining time talking and crying about his daughter, grieving her loss in a way that he had needed to protect himself from until now.

In addition to support for his walking and grief counseling, Prentice also found that training in pain-management techniques helped decrease his dependence on medication and increase his sense that he could work with, rather than against, his body.

Depression is one of the most common complaints among adults seeking psychotherapy, but it is nonetheless under-diagnosed, under-treated, and expensive (Too few people 1997). Clinical depression strikes approximately one-fifth of Americans at some point in their lives, but only 27 percent of cases receive adequate care (Rich 1997). The direct and indirect costs, financial as well as emotional, are staggering. Including treatment, premature death, absenteeism, and lost productivity, the cost may be as high as forty-three billion dollars annually (Too few people 1997). Especially with the development of new drugs, medication is often the primary means used for treating depression. Psychotherapy, whether alone or in combination with medication, is the usual alternative.

People are more aware of depression than ever before, and they're more willing to talk about it. Office visits that patients make to their doctors due to depression doubled between 1988 and 1994 (Pincus et al. 1998). Antidepressants now account for the greatest number of psychotropic drugs prescribed in the U.S.

Yet medication for depression potentially has a number of uncomfortable side effects. Among these are dizziness, sedation, dry mouth, urinary retention, weight changes, sexual dysfunction, neurological side effects, cardiovascular effects, insomnia, and anxiety (American Psychiatric Association 1993). At a time when the "explanation pendulum" for many problems has swung toward biological answers and treatments, one effective biophysical approach has been almost entirely left out of the current experimental mainstream: the use of exercise for depression, alone or in combination with psychotherapy and/or medication.

What information is available about the effectiveness of exercise when it is compared with the two major treatments, medication and psychotherapy? There has been only occasional research on this question, but in each case, exercise appears to be effective both in and of itself and in comparison to these other methods.

How Does Exercise Stack Up Against Antidepressants?

Especially since the advent of newer classes of antidepressant medication such as Prozac and other SSRIs, numerous studies of effectiveness have compared these medications with psychotherapy. But until recently, no research has examined the relative effectiveness of exercise in contrast to medication for the treatment of depression.

James Blumenthal and colleagues at Duke University have conducted a number of systematic studies of patients diagnosed with major depressive disorder using the two treatment conditions of exercise and medication. They have compared patients' response to aerobic exercise, psychotropic medication (Zoloft, an SSRI), or a combination of the two. After four and a half months of treatment, patients receiving any of these treatments were significantly less depressed. About two-thirds were no longer depressed (Blumenthal et al. 1999). These same patients were contacted six months after the original study. Patients who had been in the exercise group were more likely to be partially or fully recovered than those who were in the medication or medication plus exercise group (Babyak et al. 2000).

Some additional findings from this study are worth noting as well. In a number of situations, combining two treatments is often more effective than either alone. For example, the combination of medication *and* psychotherapy is often recommended as preferable to either alone. A case can be made, likewise, that the combination of exercise and psychotherapy may be more powerful than either alone. (See chapter 13 for more information about this.) What about the combination of exercise and medication?

Interestingly, the researchers found that the combined exercise plus medication group seemed not to do as well as the group that used exercise alone as their treatment method. The authors wondered if there may have been an "anti-medication" bias among some of the study participants. The people recruited for this research appear to have been specifically curious about the relationship between exercise and depression. Thus, those who were both exercising and taking medication might not have felt the sense of personal mastery that those using only exercise may have gained.

Almost half of the people who had participated in the medication-only group began to exercise during the six-month follow-up period. But regardless of group, the more that participants exercised, the less depressed they were.

It's clear that this is an important line of research—and that more research is needed.

How Does Exercise Compare to Therapy

At the height of the running boom, John Greist, a psychiatrist (and runner), along with a number of colleagues at the University of Wisconsin, randomly assigned twenty-eight patients seeking treatment for depression at an out-patient psychiatric clinic to three different situations: running therapy, time-limited individual psychotherapy, or time-unlimited psychotherapy (Greist et al. 1979). When checked at the end of the ten-week experiment and one and three months later, the people who ran demonstrated decreases in depression equivalent to the two psychotherapy conditions.

In a follow-up study, Klein et al. (1985) studied a larger group of depressed patients who were randomly assigned to one of four treatment conditions: running therapy, meditation/relaxation, weekly group relaxation training, and semistructured group therapy. At the end of the twelve weeks of treatment, people in each of the groups were less depressed. The improvement was somewhat stronger for those who had been in the individual instructional programs rather than the group methods. These changes were sustained over a nine-month follow-up period.

Exercise with Severely Depressed People

How effective is exercise with people who are *really* depressed? This question has not been systematically studied in North America, but some European psychiatrists have researched the topic. People hospitalized for depression tend to be inactive, and the general assumption has been that inpatients do not like strenuous exercise. Nonetheless, Norwegian psychiatrist Egil Martinsen and Dutch psychiatrist Rudi Bosscher have both noted significant improvement in hospitalized depressed patients who exercise. Martinsen even commented: "Patients evaluated physical fitness training as the most important element in the comprehensive treatment programmes. It was ranked above traditional forms of therapy: psychotherapy, milieu therapy and medication" (Martinsen 1990, p. 386). Martinsen also found that more than half the patients continued to exercise one year after termination of the formal training program. And in a recent study in Germany, twelve patients with severe depression were given a daily thirty-minute walking regime. After ten days, half of the patients were substantially less depressed—including five for whom medication had not been successful (Dimeo et al. 2001). Although a small study, this certainly supports other research in the area.

With the increasing rationing of health care, people may be markedly depressed yet not be hospitalized, or hospitalized only briefly. As recently as the mid-1990s, my client

Norman would have been hospitalized for depression. But at the time that I began working with him he wasn't considered unable to function, and so was seen on an outpatient basis.

■ Norman's Story

Norman was a gangly and disheveled fifty-three-year-old middle manager who was referred to me for psychotherapy after medication had not resolved his depression. For the past three months, he had been experiencing problems sleeping, a loss of appetite, difficulty concentrating, intense self-doubt, and uncontrollable tearfulness and emotional reactivity. This severe depression had begun and increased fairly rapidly. Otherwise, his life had been going well. He was in a comfortable marriage and had an interesting, even if moderately stressful, job.

Along with the initiation of psychotherapy, Norman started a different medication. Additionally, we discussed exercise options together. Assuming that some of the positive mental effects of exercise are biological, I thought that exercise might be especially useful for Norman. His depression appeared to be more based in his bloodstream than in external circumstances, and thus a treatment that affected his biochemistry might be especially helpful.

Norman had enjoyed roller skating in the past. Although skating at a rink wasn't convenient in his current life, he thought that in-line skating might be an attractive alternative. He bought skates and rapidly worked up to skating three to four times a week for about forty-five minutes at a time, often skating to and from work.

Some months later, as fall approached, we again reviewed Norman's exercise behaviors and plans. Ice skating or aerobics classes seemed promising possibilities during the snowy winter months.

Norman's depression gradually decreased. In order of importance, it seemed to me that the most significant factors in his improvement were: medication, exercise, and psychotherapy.

Exercise Recommendations for Lifting Your Mood

You may be experiencing temporary sadness or suffering more profound depression. How does the information in this chapter apply to you? Let's look at some practical answers.

Taking Care

Let me start these recommendations with a few important warnings that have to do with your physical as well as mental health:

1. One of the characteristics of depression is that people who are depressed often don't feel the energy to be physically active. If you're depressed, you may not currently be very active—and it may have been some time since you were.

Because of that long-term inactivity, it's especially important for you to get clearance from your health care provider before beginning an exercise program. It's likely your health care provider will be enthusiastic about this way that you're planning to take care of yourself.

2. If you are taking psychotropic medication, it will be especially important for you to review your exercise plans with your health care provider. If you've been fairly inactive, this person may suggest starting your program more slowly than if you weren't on medication—although at this point, there do not seem to be clear medical guidelines on the subject.

At fifty-seven, Rhonda has experienced depression and seasonal affective disorder (SAD) for several years. She has taken medication—and has exercised—to control the intensity of her depression:

■ Rhonda's Story

When Rhonda needed a new family doctor after her old one retired, she had a thorough physical exam and interview. Her new physician asked, among other questions, how much Rhonda exercised. A bit smug, Rhonda responded: "I walk the dog for forty-five minutes every day, and I have done yoga off and on for many years." The physician replied, "Well, with your problems, that's not enough!"

Rhonda was a bit put out. Her thought was: "Hey, I already do more regular exercise than most of my friends, and besides, my problem is a lack of energy. Whenever I have done more intensive exercise before, I have gone home exhausted and useless for several hours afterwards." But later that same week, she had an appointment with her psychiatrist. The dialogue was nearly identical. The psychiatrist told her about a new health club opening in the neighborhood and said that Rhonda should check it out. Rhonda thought, "Good grief, how can this be? I have been struggling with SAD for several years now, and no one has ever told me to get *lots* more exercise. It makes sense to churn up the endorphins, but how can I possibly do it?"

Rhonda visited the health club at the end of January. She looked at all those machines and people chugging around to the loud pounding music and thought, "Never in my wildest nightmare did I imagine myself in a gym!" But she paid the full year's fee up front, figuring that this would be an incentive to use the gym and get her money's worth. She recognized that she would need someone or something outside of herself to keep her going.

"I knew I would have to show up. I knew once I got there I would do what I had to do, but I wanted someone else firmly in charge.

"The folks at the gym were wonderful—encouraging, positive, friendly—and they've continued to be. They showed me around and introduced me to all the equipment and how to use it. Because I had no idea how to use the machines, I paid a personal trainer for one session. After taking down some information, showing me how to use the equipment, and finding out about me and my goals, she wrote out a beginning program for me. Having that plan written out really helped: I just go there and follow it. Three times a week, over the course of two hours, I do a combination of treadmill, weight machines, and yoga stretches. Since I move from cardio straight into weights straight into stretching and yoga, I don't know which is 'more' responsible for how good I feel when I leave. I know that I now would 'miss' any one component if I did a workout without it.

"I come home from a workout feeling relaxed and refreshed. I often walk to and from the gym—about a mile.

"I'm realizing that part of my emotional problems had to do with sinking self-esteem as I had gotten fatter and weaker with medication and depression. I've begun to care that my tummy sticks out, and I'm taking pride in its tightening up. I want to lose a little weight, and I feel confident that I can. I find that I have much less difficulty focusing. And I have begun to notice other things. Because I am paying attention to my body, I have noticed some days I have much more energy than others. My moods still go up and down, but now I feel good most of the time. My husband has commented on the improvement. Now that we're headed into the spring and summer seasons, I expect to feel much better anyway, but I intend to keep up the exercise routine over the summer so that I can get off to a better start next autumn and winter."

Take Your Emotional Temperature

If you're depressed, you may not be feeling especially hopeful or adventurous right now. One of the things that can be most helpful is for you to keep track of your mood both before and after you exercise. An easy way to do this is to use your Exercise Log to give yourself a rating from one to ten concerning your mood. Don't set any expectations about what your number should be, or how much it should change: just observe yourself, both before you exercise and shortly after you've finished. Notice, too, how long this mood change lasts. It's very important to *write this information down*. We all tend to forget. We all tend to minimize changes that we have made in ourselves. If you're depressed, you'll be even more likely than other people to shrug off any changes. Having this information in front of you, in black and white, will help you see that you can have some control over your mood. This attitude of curiosity lets you be that scientist or sleuth, finding out a lot about your emotions and the connections between your body and mind. Taking this one small action was the key factor in convincing Nancy of the importance of exercise for her:

■ Nancy's Story

Nancy, who is sixty-four, reluctantly dragged her previously idle treadmill out of the closet. She really didn't *like* walking. But she was a "good client," and had started this walking program because I had told her that doing some kind of exercise would be helpful—and treadmill walking seemed the most likely. Nancy began walking for fifteen minutes, two or three times a week. Carefully she rated and wrote down her mood before and after exercising. She was very surprised to see the evidence of change in her mood. She hadn't known that exercise could have that kind of impact on her. She continued to pay attention and began to notice that as the day progressed, her mood continued to improve. She recognized that if she woke up in a foul mood, walking on the treadmill turned things around. Although she couldn't schedule exercise more than three times a week, she increased the duration on the treadmill to half an hour each time.

Pay Attention to Change

As with Nancy, you may feel an immediate lift in your spirits when you exercise. If you are clinically depressed, however, it may take some months of regular exercise before you experience consistent mood elevation. For some people, the initial physical changes are more immediately pronounced. If the changes in your mood occur more gradually, you might focus on those changes that you *do* notice, such as improved physical strength and endurance—or even the fact that you are paying increased attention to taking care of yourself in healthy ways.

The Right Stuff

What kind of exercise should you do? Although most of the research on depression and exercise has been conducted with running or walking, anaerobic exercise, such as weight lifting, has also been shown to be effective. I wish I could tell you that a particular type of exercise would be just the thing to shake off those blues, that livelier is better, or that aerobics, say, would work better for you than swimming. Alas—and thank goodness—people are more complicated than that. Your task for yourself is to find out what works for you. You can find the right exercise for you through systematic experimentation.

Un-Rose Colored Glasses

One of the hazards of being depressed is that you're likely to interpret life through a negative lens. You may focus on the challenges and disappointments of situations rather than the triumphs. The following sad and frustrating story is, unfortunately, true:

◾ Glenna's Story

Thirty-two-year-old Glenna had been sinking into a continuously deeper depression over a period of weeks. As her emotional life unraveled, she found it difficult to get to work in the morning. Making meals was effortful; washing and combing her long, attractive hair became more than she could tolerate. As the weekend approached with forecasts of weather conditions ideal for skiing, we discussed ways she could cope with the weekend. An expert skier, Glenna planned a day on the slopes.

When she came in to see me early the following week, Glenna's mood, energy, and self-esteem had, if anything, sunk lower. She reported that she had spent hours cross-country skiing—and had accompanied the rhythm of the glide with the repetitive word, "Sickie, sickie, sickie." Instead of helping lift her out of her distressed mood, this potentially pleasurable and energizing time had become another way that she could beat herself up.

If, like Glenna, exercise just adds to your misery, this may be a signal that you need a major emotional overhaul. A number of self-help books can support your self-reflection and desire to think more constructively. Discussion with a therapist can give you the opportunity to observe, reflect on, and challenge your negative thoughts about yourself in the world. You may find it helpful to learn to focus on the ways in which the cup of life is half full rather than half empty. Psychotherapy can be an opportunity to share and resolve internal pain.

Making Contact

When people are depressed, they often pull back from connecting with other people. Even though you may need to push yourself a bit at first, deciding to exercise can be an opportunity for being with others. This time with other people may take the form of an actual exercise class, using the same changing room as other people and getting involved in conversation, or getting together with others in a shared activity. For example, spending time being active with other people was an important aspect of Molly's recovery.

▣ Molly's Story

At twenty-nine, Molly was granted a medical leave from work when she became overwhelmed with depression and her mental and emotional life ground to a standstill. Most days she simply lay on her bed, too tired even to read or watch TV. She was paralyzed by indecision, unable to choose what or whether to eat. Giving herself permission to eat her meals at a restaurant for a while let her feel that she was being cared for and cared about. And a few times a week, she did manage to drag herself out of her apartment to an open game of Ultimate Frisbee. Running around with a bunch of other adults—playing—took her out of herself for a few hours.

Whether or not you exercise with others, having the support of other people as you embark on exercise will be an important element for you at this time. This support may take the form of a family member who comments favorably on your increased energy or a friend who checks in (at your request!) to see if you have finally made a call to find out when the pool offers aquaerobics.

Ratcheting Up

If you've been exercising for a long time, your body may have "habituated" to the emotional effects of exercise. In that case, altering some aspect of the FIT (the frequency, intensity, or duration) of your exercise may be helpful. In particular, temporarily increasing the *intensity* of your exercise is likely to have an immediate, positive impact. Over a few weeks, increases in frequency or duration may have a positive effect as well. This particular recommendation is one that you need to monitor carefully: *overuse* of exercise (see chapter 10) can result in symptoms that look like depression. However, if you use an experimental attitude rather than a driven or compulsive approach to exercise, you will be able to differentiate whether changing the FIT is or is not helpful for you.

Just Do It

By now, the phrase "Just do it" is well-worn, yet it carries a message that is especially important if you're sad, down, or depressed, and if you are looking for a way out and a way up. Mired in your subjective experience of feeling awful, it may seem especially difficult for you to energize yourself to do anything different. Yet you know that sitting still and feeling bad leads to more sitting still and feeling bad. Movement of almost any sort gives you the opportunity to shift out of your negative mood.

Should you be highly active? Should you work out with other people? The best advice I can offer you is: Find out! Even though you are currently at an unexperimental low, try some activity, give yourself enough time to find out if it makes a difference in your mood, and keep track of what you notice about yourself. Pay attention to the vignettes in this and other chapters. These are stories of very real people, struggling with some of the same issues as you. Although it may seem effortful at first, I can almost guarantee you that, with some exploration, you will find the right kind of exercise for you.

CHAPTER 7

FEELING STRONG AND CAPABLE: SELF-ESTEEM AND COMPETENCE

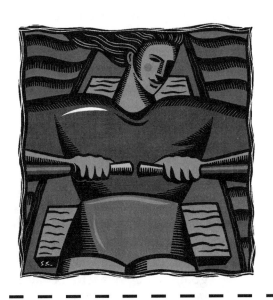

Some of us experience anxiety so challenging that it limits our ability to function, while others sail along, feeling only twinges of tension or stress. And some of us are undone by low moods and depression, while others stay fairly emotionally constant. All of us, however, come face-to-face with questions of our own self-esteem and competence. As human beings, we are uniquely hardwired to assess ourselves and our own value.

Self-esteem is described as a "multicomponent construct," a concept with many different aspects. Self-esteem relates to our capacity to function with adaptability within society and to feel in control of our lives.

People sometimes describe self-esteem as one part of our more general self-concept. Self-concept is considered "an individual's overall awareness of self in regard to physical attributes, personal characteristics, social identities, and/or behaviors" (Horn and Claytor 1993, p. 312). Self-esteem is the evaluative element of this more global self-concept. In practical terms, if self-concept refers to who we think we are, self-esteem describes how we think and feel about that self-description. Not surprisingly then, our self-esteem is closely linked to our overall sense of well-being (Sonstroem 1997). Whereas high self-esteem is generally connected to a sense of satisfaction and happiness, low self-esteem is related to depression and mental illness (Sonstroem 1997).

How does exercise fit into a discussion about self-esteem? What's the connection between exercise and self-esteem? How does our judgment of ourselves relate to our level of physical activity? The relationship between exercise and self-esteem is both intricate and important. A simplified sequence of the connection between exercise and self-esteem might look like this:

- Exercise makes you feel good,

- Feeling good increases your self-esteem,

- Therefore, exercise improves your self-esteem.

Needless to say, human beings are more complex—and less linear—than this reasoning suggests. There are various ways in which self-esteem and exercise interact. For example, physical exercise and the resulting increase in physical fitness leads to improved physical self-concept (an estimation of our physical abilities and one component of total self-esteem). In turn, improved physical self-concept leads to increased interest in physical exercise, creating a repetitive, positive loop (Sonstroem 1997). For example, I talked with thirty-three-year-old Peter about this interaction.

▪ Peter's Story

Peter wanted to decrease the performance anxiety he experienced as an actor. Particularly when preparing a script for filming or anticipating auditions, he felt paralyzed by fear that he would forget his lines.

Peter had been alcohol-free for the past four months. It was not yet his longest period of sobriety, but it was the first time that he had stopped drinking of his own accord. He understood that drinking interfered with his focused goal, which was to be acting. He was attending AA regularly and voluntarily—again, a first.

- -

EXERCISE: How Do You Affect Your Self-Esteem?

Your sense of self-esteem or competence is affected by many aspects of your daily life—what you do, what you say to yourself about yourself, how you feel, and how you interact with others. Take a moment here to reflect on those thoughts, activities, and relationships that serve to support your self-esteem and those that diminish your sense of your own competence.

Self-Esteem Enhancing Thoughts, Actions, and Relationships	*Self-Esteem Diminishing Thoughts, Actions, and Relationships*

- -

Peter had also been taking anti-anxiety medication for the past six months. He was eager to be as free of medication as he was of substances. He had already started to taper.

As we reviewed ways that Peter had coped with tension in the past, it became clear that he had used a number of effective methods in the past. He knew how to do deep, diaphragmatic breathing. He had found saunas invaluable. Though he wasn't currently exercising at all, he had run marathons a few years previously.

With a brief nudge of encouragement from me, Peter joined his local Y. He immediately embarked on a regular plan of yoga twice a week and running six miles on alternate days. Saunas were incorporated as a routine part of each visit to the Y. The results were immediate and startling.

Peter enjoyed the exercise in and of itself. He began using deep breathing before auditions and found that his attitude toward the auditions changed. For instance, after auditions he noticed himself thinking: "I did the audition as well as I could. I may or may not be the person that they pick for the part."

He also noticed that he was feeling and behaving in a less frantic way. For example, he was dissatisfied with his agent. He thought a new agent would advocate more effectively on his behalf. To prepare for this personnel change he revised his resume in a methodical manner and had new photos taken. He needed to get various pieces into place before actually sending information out to potential new agents. Earlier, he would have been scattered, getting part of the resume completed, worrying about the format, unsure about whether to get new photos or which shots to use. He would have worried, stewed, gotten started on one part, wondered who to contact—and ultimately not gotten any one piece finished. We discussed the ways in which he was putting into practice the AA philosophy of taking action about the things he could control and letting go of those that he couldn't.

I asked Peter to notice what he was thinking about and saying to himself as he ran. Over and over, no matter how he thought or what the topic was, he said that he ended up with a feeling of confidence. Whether at his part-time job or in relation to his acting work, this sense of capability allowed him to approach situations with a new level of ease. This comfort with himself in turn helped him feel more confident and competent.

Feeling Good About Yourself

The interaction between exercise and self-esteem can occur in relation to many aspects of ourselves. We'll focus here on skill, competence, body image, and optimism.

— —

EXERCISE: MINING THE SYMBOLISM

Exercise contains many opportunities to symbolically represent the relationship between what we are actually doing and how we're experiencing it. How does the physical strength you derive from exercise assist you in understanding your own mental and emotional strength or power? Circle those words that describe the ways in which your body assists you in becoming more conscious of yourself—and add some of your own.

Able	Powerful
Active	Skillful
Competent	Strong
Courageous	
Energetic	Substantive
In balance	Solid
Persistent	Other: _____

— —

Doing Good and Feeling Capable

Self-esteem is related to both our sense of how skilled we are and how competent we feel. In another chicken-and-egg loop, as we develop more skill there is an improvement in our self-esteem, and as our self-esteem improves our openness to skill-building increases. If we apply this loop to exercise, we notice that as we become more skilled physically, there is an increase in self-esteem. Likewise, as we feel better about our physical skill, our performance skill increases.

Like the chicken and the egg, it doesn't matter which comes first. But significantly, the research shows that it's not the *actual* increase in fitness that increases self-esteem as much as people's *perceptions* of their improvement (Sonstroem 1997).

Who gains the most in self-esteem when exercising? Gains in self-esteem through exercise are greater for those with initially lower self-esteem scores, as well as those with lower fitness who value an increase in some aspect of fitness or skill. Research suggests that these increases in self-esteem are relatively long-lasting.

Other aspects of self-esteem involve a sense of competence, mastery, or self-sufficiency, and a broadened or increased sense of identity. These again are key factors in exercise. Johnsgard (1989) suggests that when we exercise, we may develop an internal sense of: "No doctors. No pills. I did it. I know how. I could do it again" (p. 50). As we mentioned in chapter 6, the mood improvement for the exercising subjects in Blumenthal's depression studies may derive at least in part from just this sense of personal accomplishment. Our changed self-concept reflects the sense that "in addition to whatever else I may be, I am a physically active person." Exercise becomes more important, and the *self* becomes more important.

Exercise can also enhance or underscore those aspects of ourselves that are important to us. Carolyn, now fifty-eight, has taken great pride in her gardening for many years.

■ Carolyn's Story

Although she loved gardening, finding infinite variety in flowers and vegetables, Carolyn also recognized the toll that the bending and lifting took on her body. She would pay for an hour in the garden with two hours of discomfort.

Carolyn started going to a local gym to counteract the continuous effects of gravity and age: she read an article that convinced her that strengthening her muscles and heart was the only way that she might prevent the ongoing "spreading" of her body that so distressed her. With brief input from a trainer, she developed a routine that included weight training alternating with cardiovascular activity, and she surprised herself by discovering that she enjoyed the peace and solitude she experienced at the gym.

A few months into her new program, gardening season brought another unanticipated but significant reward and reinforcement. The movements that had been so wearing and exhausting the prior year now felt effortless. Her pleasure in the beauty of her creation served to support a sense of the power and beauty of the human body at work in its own growth and creation.

Outer Reflections of Inner Mirrors

Body image is another element in the interaction between self-esteem and exercise. Regardless of gender, dissatisfaction with body image is correlated with low self-esteem, insecurity, and depression (Rejeski and Thompson 1993). Exercise, on the other hand, changes what your body actually looks like. Your strengthened muscles and bodily tone and your reconfigured body shape bring you back to the body that you were designed to have in the first place. Exercise is infinitely less expensive than nipping and tucking—and utterly more natural. The literal changes in how our bodies look with exercise are reflected in our mental and emotional response to these changes. Now that he is forty, my colleague and friend Steve can reflect on his history of exercise and his sense of his body:

▣ Steve's Story

Steve described himself as frequently ill when he was young, "the epitome of the ninety-pound weakling. I hated gym class, in part because of my general lack of competence, but also because I was often harassed in the locker room by classmates and in class by coaches. (Perhaps they knew I was gay before I did.) I used to joke about being the model for the "before" pictures in advertisements for exercise equipment—though it didn't feel very funny. I gave up on sports in junior high after being ridiculed by a coach for being the last one to finish a one-mile run."

In college, Steve took some aerobics classes, and then some years later began running as a way to deal with stress and clear his head after work. He jogged a mile or two a few days a week. At thirty-seven, Steve joined the Frontrunners, a gay running group. He soon realized that if he were going to keep up with the group, he'd have to develop better stamina. He increased his mileage dramatically and finished his first marathon two years later.

"It wasn't until I trained for the marathon that I began to experience the physical and psychological benefits of running longer distances. A couple of miles a day had helped me deal with stress, but the distances and commitment required in training for a marathon changed the way I felt about my body and the way I thought about myself. For the first time in my life, I liked the way my body felt and looked."

Steve's story is interesting for a number of reasons. He used exercise as a method of stress management. But the change in his sense of self seems to have occurred once he dramatically increased the entire FIT (frequency, intensity, and time) of the exercise that he was doing. The sense of friendship and identity with other members of this particular group may have also been an element in his changed body image and self-esteem.

Exercise and Optimism

Exercise is related to a general sense of well-being and optimism. Research suggests that people who exercise regularly are found to be generally more optimistic. Kavussanu and McAuley (1995) concluded that people who are typically apprehensive may decrease their sense of general concern when they exercise. Their positive outlook comes from a sense of mastery or accomplishment as a result of activity. Alternatively, a positive sense of self may lead people to engage in health-promoting behaviors which result in a sense of well-being. In either event, there seem to be long-lasting as well as short-term positive effects.

Exercise Recommendations

As with stress and depression, there is no one "right" form of exercise to increase self-esteem. Nonetheless, we can offer some specific tips.

Rating without Judging

Can you evaluate yourself without making judgments about yourself? I've suggested using a mental 1 to 10 scale to measure your "before" and "after" experience of anxiety and depression in relation to exercise. You can use this same internal measurement in relation to what you think of yourself or how you feel about yourself. Before exercising and shortly after exercising, assign yourself a number (and record it!) to represent your sense of self-esteem or competence. See whether there are short-term or immediate effects, or if self-esteem changes are more gradual, such that your rating change is noticeable only over time.

Being Strong and Feeling Strong

For people in general and women in particular, the physical strength increase that accompanies weight lifting can translate symbolically into a psychological sense of increased strength. Karen Andes' book, *A Woman's Book of Strength: An Empowering Guide to Total Mind/Body Fitness* (1995), provides both important understandings of the link between physical and emotional strength and practical information on strength training.

My thirty-year-old client Nicole has experienced this real and symbolic effect at various points in her life.

▣ *Nicole's Story*

In college, Nicole played varsity volleyball, but then a chronic lower-back problem brought a four-year halt to her exercising. Two years ago, shortly after she and her boyfriend broke up, Nicole decided it was time to feel better about herself and get back into the shape she wanted to be in, so she joined a gym and began weight training.

She started slowly, frustrated that she couldn't lift the weights she had previously, though she knew that would come with time. "As the months went by, and I got into better shape, my friends and family began to notice the definition and muscle tone. The strength I felt was not restricted to the physical: I was becoming more self-confident and assertive, and the people around me noticed this change as well.

"And then, about a year ago, I just lost the mental ability to do strength training. I knew something was wrong with me, but I couldn't figure it out. I could not motivate myself into that gym to do a weight program. I could go in and do a cardio workout every day, but weights suddenly felt beyond my ability."

Two months later, Nicole experienced complete "burnout" at work and in her whole life. Although she still liked being active, the rhythm and discipline of weight lifting seemed beyond her. As she began to recover, she thought that she could resume weight training. For a while, getting herself to do the weight training once a week was all she could manage. Again, she felt disheartened, realizing that she'd lost so much ground, yet she recognized that once a week was a start. At least she was a few steps ahead of where she had been for the past several months.

"A few weeks ago, I experienced the most motivating sign that I was finally back on track with my life and 'normal' activities for me. It was the day I realized that I really wanted to do the weights. That realization alone was astounding. I sat there at the squat rack, looking at how far I had come in the past year. Full circle, in a sense. What was meaningful was not only my desire to take part in the weight-training session, but also what it meant in my recovery. I needed to have psychological and emotional strength in order to do the weight training. I knew I had come back to myself.

"Weight training not only shapes your physical body, but also reflects your inner strength. It takes that inner strength to get yourself motivated to go to the gym to train and to sustain you through a challenging session. The weights take strength and give you strength.

"I have a real sense of pride in myself internally, knowing how far I've come. And there's a secondary motivator: I feel proud of how I look. I feel confident in myself and my appearance."

Acknowledging Our Own Rights and Needs

When regular exercise is incorporated into your sense of self, you may notice a shift in your awareness of the importance of meeting your own psychobiological needs. Johnsgard (1989) comments: "When we begin to exercise every day, insist that an hour of each day belongs to ourselves exclusively, and tell others that they will have to somehow adjust their needs and expectations to allow us our exercise period, we're making a strong statement about ourselves: 'My running is important. My time is important. My needs are important. I am important'" (p. 50). Truly accepting and asserting this self-directed statement then gives us strength and energy to be open to and give to others. Instead of a sense of entitlement, a disregard for others and their needs, this awareness can give us additional appreciation of and ability to respond to the balanced needs of all.

Celebrate Persistence

If you want to increase your self-esteem through exercise, it's important to focus in particular on success experiences, your feelings of increased physical competence, and goal attainment. Regular journaling and occasional reflection support this aspect of well-being. Being particularly conscious of the persistence that it takes to exercise and the positive outcomes that result can help reinforce exercise and support your sense of competence and self-esteem. The positive effects of exercise will be increased if you anticipate and attribute changes to exercise and mastery.

CHAPTER 8

THE POETRY OF THE SUNRISE: CLEAR AND CREATIVE THINKING

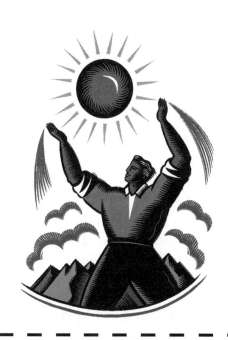

At this point we've looked at the ways that exercise is an important and effective method of dealing with various mental or emotional problems and distresses. And we've reviewed the ways in which exercise can play a useful role in building up and maintaining your positive sense of self. But there's more! In fact, one of the best kept secrets is that exercise helps you think clearly and feel connected with the world.

Why is this particular exercise effect so little known? Well, because these thoughts and feelings are very difficult to measure. In fact, as you'll see, they seem to share some of the qualities of dream states. Much of what we do know is from anecdotes and descriptions that people have shared. You'll hear a number of voices in this chapter—mostly from colleagues of mine whose attitudes and experiences I've surveyed. I hope you will use these descriptions as a sort of guide into noticing similar kinds of experiences that you may have when exercising.

This clarity of thinking and capacity to synthesize in new ways is a phenomenon that may be particularly accessible to us either while we're active or within a short time afterward. The shift in thinking is rarely described, defined, or commented upon—and it's notoriously challenging to researchers (Sachs 1984). The ways in which this increased productivity and creativity might enhance the therapeutic process have only occasionally been explored (Murphy 1996).

People rarely *begin* exercising for these effects. But for a number of people, this cognitive component becomes an integral aspect to exercise maintenance. Knowing more about what exercise can do for you will add to your interest in exercise initiation and maintenance while giving you a wider repertoire of possible uses for exercise.

Although these topics are really all interwoven and don't separate out neatly, we'll cluster the discussion into focus on thinking, creativity, peak moments or "flow," and more mystical feelings related to awe and our relationship with the universe.

Moving Your Body and Your Mind: Exercise and Thinking

Studies of thinking and exercise have focused primarily on changes in thinking in relation to aging. For example, among other conclusions of the Duke Aging and Exercise Study (a series of research projects on the subject), recent findings suggest that exercise has a direct impact on our thinking, improving our mental sharpness and skills. After four months of aerobic exercise, participants in one study had improved their performance on tests of memory and some of the more complex thought processes, such as planning and organizing tasks (Khatri et al. 2001).

In a naturalistic review (rather than an experiment) of people's lives, a recent national study of 4,600 Canadians age sixty-five or older found that, over a five year period, those who exercised were less likely to develop mental impairments associated with aging, including Alzheimer's disease. Even though *any* level of exercise seemed to provide a protective function, the more that people exercised, the less likely they were to suffer from mental declines. Those who exercised vigorously at least three times a week had the lowest risk of developing Alzheimer's (Laurin et al. 2001).

Even with younger people, exercise is associated with clear thinking. A meta-analysis (an analysis of the studies) of 134 studies of exercise and cognitive functioning reviewed tasks including reaction time, memory, reasoning, and academic achievement tests in relation to exercise. A small but significant improvement in cognitive functioning was noted (Etnier et al. 1997).

Just as we have come to understand our minds and bodies as fully interrelated, exercise has the capacity to integrate all aspects of our thinking. Active people report the experience of increased access to their mental processes. For example, people sometimes talk about "right brain" and "left brain" thinking, and though there are various centers for all different kinds of thinking throughout the brain, this differentiation can be a simplified method of categorizing some aspects of our thinking. In this understanding, "left brain" thinking is linear, analytic, and static. "Right brain" thinking, on the other hand, is described as integrative, intuitive, and holistic. Both are important to our daily lives; each is especially important to some kinds of mental processing. Part of what happens during exercise is that for some people the "right brain" functions become more accessible than in everyday life. Greater accessibility means that this mode of thinking can become available to our more organized and systematic thinking functions. For lack of a better term, we can describe this synthesis as "right brain problem solving." A friend and colleague, a forty-seven-year-old psychologist named Doug, experienced the pleasure of using exercise for thinking:

■ Doug's Story

He said that his long, slow distance runs were a "personal treasure." Although he occasionally would run with others, he preferred running alone. He used the time during the run as a primary opportunity for reflection and planning. He commented that he had outlined entire articles and presentations in his head during a single run.

Doug described this mental experience as similar to hypnotic trance. "I play with the ideas, allow my thoughts to drift in various directions and then focus back to the theme at hand. In retrospect it is a flowing process between both convergent and divergent thinking. While I might be able to duplicate the process in non-exercise settings, the distractions and demands of other contexts would serve as major obstacles."

Exercise and Creativity

The integration of "right" and "left" brain thinking reaches full flower when we look at creativity. And exercise can be the nourishment that helps that flower bloom. There seems to be a pattern linking exercise to increased creativity, although this connection is more anecdotal than based on research. If studies on exercise and thinking could be described as sparse, those on creativity and exercise are nearly nonexistent. And yet, the phenomenon is there. Even someone as frequently inarticulate as President George W. Bush was able to describe the connection between the familiar surroundings of his Texas ranch, being outside in companionable solitude with his dogs, and the rhythmic repetitiveness of movement that provided the setting for the development of his inaugural speech:

> Anyway, it's kind of neat to go out there, the sun was beginning to rise, and play with the little guy [his dog]. It's beautiful kind of pasture. Then I went for a run with the other dog and just walked. And I started thinking about a lot of things. I was able to—I can't remember what it was. Oh, the inaugural speech, started thinking through that. (*US News and World Report* 2001, p. 17)

The characteristics of aerobic exercise that Berger (1994) describes as essential to mood improvement—rhythmic, repetitive activity that needs little concentration in and of itself—may be those that also allow the mind to drift, yet in a very focused way. Exercise that is repetitive and rhythmical, often exercise that occurs within a defined space, seems to encourage introspection or creative thinking. Perhaps it's the repetitive monotony of the movements, the solitude that's often involved, the diaphragmatic breathing that accompanies the activity—or some combination of these. It is almost a hypnotic effect that allows for wide-ranging thoughts, reflection, and creativity. There is a sense of order that has much more of the intuitive, holistic, all-encompassing sweep than of a linear, hierarchical sequence. "The routine rhythmic motion of running or walking, in particular, requires little thought or attention. Anyone who has run or walked regularly for even a few minutes knows how the mind seems to open to a flood of thoughts and emotions; solutions to nagging problems suddenly appear like flashing 100-watt bulbs" (Paffenbarger and Olsen 1996, p. 225).

Neurologist and author Oliver Sacks describes his own experience in regard to swimming:

> There was a total engagement in the act of swimming, in each stroke, and at the same time the mind could float free, become spellbound, in a state like a trance. . . . There is something about being in water and swimming which alters my mood, gets my thoughts going, as nothing else can. Theories and stories would construct themselves in my mind as I swam to and fro, or round and round. . . . Sentences and paragraphs would write themselves in my mind, and at such times I would have to come to shore every so often to discharge them. (1997, p. 45)

Joyce Carol Oates, the prolific novelist, uses running for a variety of purposes: running has been the place and the space where she has created parts of various novels, later transcribing the imagery and thoughts that emerged while running. And she points to poet Walt Whitman's long walks, reflected in the rhythm of his poetry.

Nietzsche commented that the best thoughts come while walking. Ever on the alert for this connection, George Sheehan wrote: "Somehow, running gives me the word, the phrase, the sentence that is just right" (1978, p. 15). And alert as well for others who made a similar connection, Sheehan often cited Henry David Thoreau, a "great walker," as an example of someone who took advantage of the mind-body connection through exercise. Sheehan quotes Thoreau: "I inhabit my body with inexpressible satisfaction: both its weariness and its refreshments," and comments, "Thoreau's other activities derived their vitality from the vitality of his body" (1978, p. 52). (As if to underscore this point, sections of this book—some of the word play and parts of this chapter in particular—have "shown up" in my head as I was swimming, as well as on first awakening in the morning.)

This intimate relationship between movement and creativity led Julia Cameron, who has written a number of well-known books on "the artist within," to recommend rhythmic, repetitive forms of exercise as a necessary component to liberating the artistic, creative self that resides within people (1992). "We learn to look at things with a new perspective. . . . Seemingly without effort, our answers come while we swim or stride or ride or run" (Cameron 1992, p. 189).

When is this kind of thinking most effective? Often it's most powerful when you feel at a dead end with straightforward, linear, "left brain" thinking. Some issues are too large for a single sequence of thought to encompass them. Other concerns need a new approach, a different angle. These are the perfect moments for "taking your thoughts for a run." There are various ways to do this: one is to ask yourself a significant question and then deliberately *not* think about it while exercising. A solution or a new approach may emerge. The background work was occurring while you were exercising. Alternatively, a forty-two-year-old psychologist colleague, Amanda, uses her exercise time to focus on specific issues:

■ *Amanda's Story*

Amanda describes the thinking that occurs when she is jogging as both "free" and very creative. Although she says she has no idea where some of these thoughts come from, she has developed a method for tapping into this thought process: "If I want a new idea about something or want to solve a problem, I'll bring my focus back to the topic, gently ask myself to think about it, and let my thoughts wander. When I realize I'm off the topic, I gently return my focus to the topic—or explode with some new idea altogether."

This kind of thinking seems linked to the intuitive, creative, "right brain" thinking that happens in dream states. Like dreaming, these thoughts and conclusions can be highly playful. You need to treat these thoughts with respect however: like dream states, they are fragile and fluid. If you don't write down at least a corner of what your thought was, it can vanish as quickly as it miraculously appeared.

Karen, a forty-one-year-old psychologist, shared her experiences with me. The process of "cognitive clarity" was part of what was so compelling for her:

■ *Karen's Story*

Karen commented that her mind gets clear of much of its clutter with exercise, allowing her to focus on issues and ideas. Her mental pace slows down. She feels no need to solve anything, but rather senses that she can just be present with her thoughts. The typical consequence is that she experiences very clear and powerful insights regarding problems, solutions, and new ideas.

"There is a qualitative aspect to this process. I feel like I get in touch with my whole being—with the world. I leave logic and analytical thinking behind. I sit with the process of life, which to me is more qualitative in nature."

Once you have experienced and practiced this kind of thinking, you can set the stage for it to appear at your bidding. Regardless of the activity, Tory, a forty-four-year-old psychologist friend and colleague finds this particular space for herself:

◼ *Tory's Story*

Depending on the time of year, Tory may be involved in one or another sport. She actively seeks out the creative possibilities that come alive for her with activity. She told me:

"Mostly I create, write, go into this world of ideas which is so magical in that it has no relation to the troubles of my world or personal life. Sometimes I space out on the scenery, especially if I go skiing alone. Other times I tune into the power of my physical self. But I always go somewhere great and seem to know how to get there. Sometimes it happens the moment I don the shoes and head out the door to run or slip on my goggles to swim along the lap lane. Other times, I breathe into it and the magic appears."

And another colleague and friend, Charles, a forty-year-old psychologist, elaborated on the ways in which this type of thinking shares a relationship with dreaming:

◼ *Charles' Story*

It's this effortless "dream thinking," as Charles describes it, that he finds so intriguing. He recognizes that it is the way that human beings usually process information, even though education and graduate school training are designed to shape our thinking in a rational, conscious, and linear manner. We've just learned to ignore and devalue the more fluid state.

"On long runs I seem to be able to pull together information in novel ways, by letting go of consciously linear thinking patterns. On the surface, these might appear as random thoughts, yet they end up coming together in delightful and meaningful ways. For example, I come up with some of my best paper and presentation titles while running. The problem is, of course, in order to use any of these great ideas you have to remember them long enough to get through the rest of the run and get back to a pen and paper.

"This is the same thing that happens in dreams. You wake up from a dream that gives you obvious insight but don't think to write it down—you say, it was so powerful you'll never forget—then the next morning you no longer have the access code! I've learned—the hard way—to write down those great ideas."

Going with the Flow

As with some other activities, you may experience peak moments when you exercise. These go by different names, depending on the person doing the labeling and/or the activity. The terms "flow," "exercise high," or being "in the zone" are commonly used. People have experienced the "runner's high" frequently enough that the term is specifically attributed to that sport. These feeling states are not necessarily the same as peak *performance*, which really reflects superior or outstanding behavior. Instead, this sensation of flow is an emotional and psychological experience.

Regardless of the activity, people who experience this phenomenon frequently describe common specific elements, such as the merging of action and awareness; a sense of balance between challenge and skill; loss of self-consciousness; and the transformation of time. Mihalyi Csikszentmihalyi, a psychologist at the University of Chicago who has studied flow for many years, describes this phenomenon as an optimal state "in which people are so involved in an activity that nothing else seems to matter; the experience itself is so enjoyable that people will do it even at great cost, for the sheer sake of doing it" (1990, p. 4). The runner's high may be a specific type of peak experience, characterized by euphoria, a heightened sense of well-being, feelings of psychological/physical strength and power, a glimpse of perfection, and even spirituality (Berger 1996).

Csikszentmihalyi describes the activity of flow:

> Although the flow experience appears to be effortless, it is far from being so. It often requires strenuous physical exertion, or highly disciplined mental activity. It does not happen without the application of skilled performance. Any lapse in concentration will erase it. And yet while it lasts consciousness works smoothly, action follows action seamlessly. In normal life, we keep interrupting what we do with doubts and questions. "Why am I doing this? Should I perhaps be doing something else?" Repeatedly we question the necessity of our actions, and evaluate critically the reasons for carrying them out. But in flow there is no need to reflect, because the action carries us forward as if by magic. (1990, p. 54)

How many people experience this kind of ecstasy through exercise? Reports range widely. It is challenging to measure and it's elusive: if you actively try to create a peak moment, you probably won't experience it. By definition, this sense of ecstasy tends to be unplanned and arises spontaneously.

What you can do, however, is create the opportunity for this kind of experience. Not surprisingly, many of the characteristics needed to achieve flow are the qualities that allow for the optimal mental benefits of exercise. Thus, flow is likely to occur with rhythmic, repetitive exercise. For some people, length of time (exercising for a longer period of time) is a significant factor. Being alone or alone with your thoughts allows you to turn deeply inward.

And like an awake and aware dream state, this access to the inner reaches of your being can provide rich and profound understandings of yourself and the world. The irony and wonder of flow is that, as a human being, all that you can do is set the stage for this phenomenon to occur within you—and exercise is one means for doing that.

Stillness in Motion: Exercise and Mystical Awe

Indian yoga master B.K.S. Iyengar has said, "The body is the surface of the mind, and the mind is the surface of the soul." Are there truly ways in which one can experience awe through exercise? Again, this intangible but real experience is part of what holds some people to exercise. The sense of communion with the universe that many people gain through movement is powerful and healing. These mystical moments of ecstasy or a sense of awe and appreciation for the mystery of the universe, are sensations that can emerge from various activities (Csikszentmihalyi 1990; Murphy and White 1995).

For some people, it is the letting go of thought, truly *being* in the experience, that creates the sense of fullness and oneness with the world.

Claudia, a thirty-four-year-old social worker, has used running to play with her own thinking patterns.

■ Claudia's Story

As she begins her morning run during the work week, Claudia's initial thoughts relate to work issues and dilemmas. Jogging at a pace that feels comfortable for her body and mind on that particular day, these thoughts run their course in short order. She sets minigoals for the workout. Her mind turns to enjoying the technical aspects, improving her running form, lengthening her stride, increasing the cadence, and so on. Claudia begins thinking inward to the rhythm of her heart, lungs, and muscles. She is aware of the sensation of sweat. She usually takes routes that have the least traffic and most natural environment, off-road when possible. These paths and trails augment access to the sensory experience of the world around her—smells, sounds, trees, birds, and wind.

Claudia's description of her experience illustrates the gentle weaving of mind and body, thought, feeling, and meditation:

"When I'm exercising, my thinking is less task-oriented, less 'tight,' and much more meditative and sensory-involved. I enjoy the meditative state of exercise, with thoughts nowhere in particular but roaming in free and released fashion. This is often a time of simply 'coming to terms' with feelings and situations. But this does not mean it is not focused—the mind-body connection is stronger. I think about and visualize my goals, and they happen. It's very hypnotic or zen-like when things are going well. Even on days when it is harder to relax and get into the rhythm of the workout, I usually find at the end, when I stop or return to work, that I experienced some meditative level that clearly nourished me. I find that I meet frustration in my exercise routine only when I try to push to do an external goal rather than the level of activity that feels right at that moment."

The circumstances that may open you to a sense of oneness with the universe are similar to those that allow for the emergence of creativity or flow. Perhaps more than with those others, activity that occurs out-of-doors seems to be especially conducive to the sense of awe.

EXERCISE: Accessing Your Mind Through Exercise

Which aspects of this kind of thinking intrigue you—problem solving, creativity, flow, or awe? With the examples of others' voices clear in your head, use this space to discover your own voice. Keep track of external facts that seem related to increased access to your right brain thinking, for example: the type of exercise, intensity, length of time, time of day, or location that were in effect when you had the experience.

Note whether you've given yourself specific instructions. You may decide to think deliberately about an issue or you may set the stage and then *not* think about it directly. Alternatively, you may choose to open your mind and your sensory awareness to whatever may come.

Date	External Facts	Instructions	Outcome
_____	_____	_____	_____
_____	_____	_____	_____
_____	_____	_____	_____
_____	_____	_____	_____
_____	_____	_____	_____
_____	_____	_____	_____
_____	_____	_____	_____
_____	_____	_____	_____
_____	_____	_____	_____

JOURNAL TASK: EXERCISE THINKING

If this aspect of exercise interests and motivates you, make liberal use of the "Comments" column in your ongoing Exercise Log.

Having understood the methods and applications of exercise for mental well-being, we will pay particular attention to the maintenance of your momentum. In part III, we'll explore issues of ongoing motivation, as well as some of the complexities of the connections between mental functioning and exercise.

PART 3

"NOW WHAT?" MAINTAINING YOUR GAINS

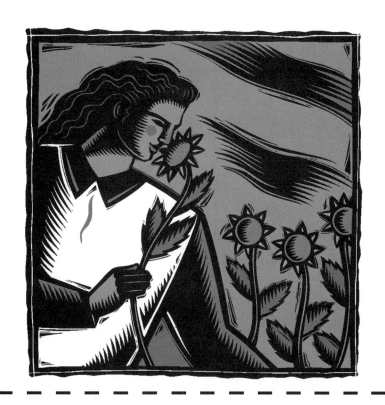

Chapter 9

Keeping Going . . . and Getting Going Again

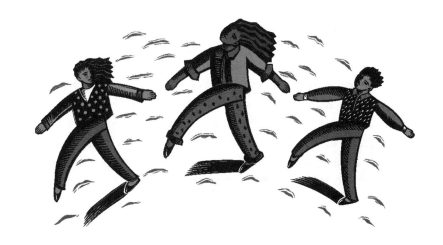

Hopefully, you've hit upon the "just right exercise," and you experience no difficulty adhering to your exercise goals. You may have made the right guess about what will work for you. Perhaps you've learned from past experience. Maybe serendipity happened. Whatever the reason, there is a fairly immediate link between you and this form of exercise. When that occurs, the issue of motivation becomes irrelevant: the exercise itself provides all the reinforcement that you need to keep going. Barring major problems, the habit is well on its way to being established. For you, there is a deep sense of pleasure, an interaction of challenge, expectation, clear feedback, focused attention, and absorption in the activity.

Enjoyment or intrinsic or internal motivation is a central aspect that affects exercise adherence and improved psychological well-being. I have to admit to being one of those "overnight converts," and no one could have been more surprised than I. In my late thirties I began running. Before then, I certainly knew other people who ran—even some of my best friends. But I truly didn't "get" it. Why, I wondered, did they arise early in the morning? Why did they engage in this repetitive, boring activity day after day?

A friend and I went out for a walk one evening in May. In New Hampshire, May is black fly season, the time when "no-seeums" swarm and nip at every unprotected part of your anatomy. Our conversation was intense but not strong enough to overcome the distraction of being bitten. We parted company. Anne went home, and I started running, so that I could get away from the flies and tolerate being outdoors a while longer. I ran perhaps two telephone pole lengths and then, out of breath, I walked for a while. It had felt good, so I ran a small distance again and then walked for a while.

I didn't give the evening's events much thought—until the next evening. I had the sensation that my body was "speaking" to me, telling me to try this activity again. And I've been running ever since.

I learned a lot from that experience. For one, running helped me through a difficult personal time in my life. Also, I learned to trust the insights and new understandings that occurred to me when I ran. I became interested in sport psychology, this field that addresses the relationship between the body and the mind through physical activity. And I learned that you can't always predict which form of exercise will be the one that has sustaining power for you. What may appear boring from the outside can be experienced as utterly fascinating from within. This intrinsic motivation is what will keep you going in the long run.

Many people—probably most—don't experience the "aha!" of exercise right away. And for many, even if we do experience it, it isn't with the first form of exercise we try or the first time we try it. Although I gave a snapshot of myself above, my introduction to running certainly wasn't the first time I'd ever intentionally exercised. I'd just never been able to stay with it before then. For most of us, sticking with the plan can often be an issue. Predictably, 50 percent of people stop exercising within six months of beginning an exercise program (Dishman 1988). This statistic is not really as alarming as it appears, since this 50 percent adherence/50 percent dropout rate is similar to that for any health behavior change.

Reprise

Have you ever listened to a musical, whether at the theatre, on film, or on CD? After the plot has been laid out, songs that you heard before will be repeated in a slightly different way. They help move the plot along. These earlier melodies, back once again, are "reprised." Maintenance of behavior change is kind of like a reprise. Our discussion here will bring back in some familiar themes, geared toward assisting you in continuing to move (your body and your mind, if not the plot!).

If you've begun exercising, what can you do in order to continue and sustain your activity so that you move from the Action mode of behavior change to that of Maintenance? We spoke about Maintenance briefly, in chapter 3, but it's such an important part of this undertaking that it deserves more thorough discussion.

Your Attitude of Curiosity

Your attitude of curiosity or experimentation continues to be a central aspect of this exercise adventure. Are you seeing your curious self more as a metaphorical "scientist" or a "detective"? At this point in your exercise and mental health quest, what have you learned? What methods have you developed for understanding more about yourself?

The energy that you put into understanding yourself and your body-mind functioning serves to keep you interested in this ongoing process. And that interest serves to reinforce and sustain your work on this new way of behaving and understanding yourself.

Monitoring and Logging: Themes and Variations

Once you're exercising regularly, one of the most important ways that you can strengthen your exercise pattern is by developing a system to monitor your exercise. Record keeping is both a reinforcer and a basis for information—about what you've done, what you've thought, and what you will choose to do in the future. I hope that by now you've discovered the value of keeping a record for yourself.

I've been championing the idea of your keeping an exercise journal, which we're calling an Exercise Log. Here's what's vital: that you keep some kind of record. Here's what's less important: what the particular record looks like. Record keeping may involve a chart, a log, or a narrative diary. It can be simple or complex. Your log can serve as a source of motivation, a method of immediate and positive reinforcement, a chronicle of progress, a location for problem description and resolution, and an indication of program adherence. Human memory is both objectively and subjectively imperfect, and so a written record serves as a sentinel of reality. Perhaps you feel you haven't accomplished much. You've walked briskly for "only" fifteen minutes. Yet if you look back at your own record, you can see that two weeks ago you felt winded after an effortful ten minutes of walking.

If you decide not to use the Exercise Log, you can still keep very simple yet meaningful records of the exercise that you do. If you want to keep track of frequency, a check mark on your wall calendar is perfectly acceptable. If you do more than one kind of exercise, you could indicate frequency and type by using a capital letter to record the kind of exercise you did on that day. Time or duration, similarly, can be indicated just by noting the number of minutes. Some people choose to get "high tech" about it:

■ *James' Story*

James uses his new "toy," his Palm Pilot, to keep track of his yoga practice. When he takes a yoga class, he writes in "Y*ga." The yoga process and sense of body ease is so satisfying that he's started regularly doing some of his favorite yoga stretches before getting dressed in the morning. He writes in "y*" to mark these shorter segments. When he wants to review his overall frequency, he taps the "Find" indicator and writes in "y*." Milliseconds later, he has a full display of all of the yoga in which he is engaged.

Alternatively, you can go low tech:

■ *Rebecca's Story*

Thirty-eight-year-old Rebecca has kept a journal for years. When she started running, she created a pictorial shorthand for herself that became part of her ongoing narrative journal. She used long lines to indicate running and short dashes to describe walking. As she began running more of the time and walking less, the lines without breaks were an indicator to her of her increasing stamina.

- -

EXERCISE: MODIFYING MY EXERCISE LOG

Now that you've been keeping your Exercise Log for a while, what modifications make sense to you? How much time do you actually take to track your exercise behaviors and your thoughts? How do you use the information? Describe some changes that you want to incorporate into your journaling:

_____

_____

_____

When will you review and evaluate these modifications? _____

What will your criteria be? _____

_____

- -

Motivation—and Goal Setting—Revisited

Motivation for exercise often changes over time. Reviewing and reflecting on the "why" of your exercising can be a way to maintain momentum. Take, for example, running. Some years ago, Keith Johnsgard, a psychologist in California, surveyed a number of long-time runners. Although there were some gender differences in motive, Johnsgard found that

> being lean and fit become taken for granted—accomplishments which will persist as a part of a new lifestyle. . . . As . . . [the] weeks roll by, psychological benefits are realized and become central motives. These increasingly strong motives have to do with how we feel about ourselves and with how we feel, our emotional moods. They become basic in sustaining regular training for both sexes (1989, p. 49).

Goal Setting

Goal setting is useful in getting started on your exercise program. For exercise maintenance, goal review is essential. This may be a formal review or an informal reflection. Various aspects of goal setting and review were described in chapter 3, when we first looked at exercise initiation: SMART (specific, measurable, action-oriented, realistic, and timed) goals, multiple goals, and both short- and long-term goals. Just as your motivation may shift over time, your goals may, as well. Your goals may involve change, improvement, or accomplishment. The competition "bug" may bite. Or your goals may reflect an intention to maintain: to keep exercising for as long in your life as you possibly can. As Ashley Montagu commented, "The idea is to die young, as late as possible."

At eighty-six, Randall continues to exercise regularly.

■ *Randall's Story*

Randall described a weekly schedule of thirty minutes of swimming, five or six times a week, plus a mile-long walk three times a week. Ten years ago, he still lifted weights, but ultimately he decided that for him it was swimming that provided the best "feel good" experience. He commented that if he doesn't exercise, he feels slowed down and apathetic, even at times a little depressed. And he mentioned, further:

"Exercise makes my life ever so much more enjoyable. I feel more optimistic. After my swim, I want to (and sometimes do) sing, 'It's a wonderful world.' Even though she's heard me say it dozens of times, when I leave the swim club, I sometimes say to the lady at the desk, 'I feel seventy again.' She always smiles."

The goal setting described thus far refers to the "what" of exercise, but goals can also reflect the "why" of exercise. People often set health-related goals initially. But non-health related goals, such as developing recreational skills, social relationships, and satisfying one's curiosity, are the ones that seem to keep people coming back for more.

Those are the kind of goals that seem to be important to people who continue exercising throughout their lives.

As you become more aware of the variety of psychological benefits of exercise, you can have greater flexibility in using exercise to suit your own purpose. Sally began running for weight management but kept at it for all of the additional positive effects she discovered.

■ Sally's Story

As Sally's body shape began to change (more than her weight), she took her body measurements and wrote down those numbers in her journal every few weeks. In her diary, she recorded random thoughts and insights that occurred during her run in a different colored ink so that she could see them easily whenever she wanted to find them. She hadn't really understood about the stress-reducing effects of exercise, but quickly discovered that running helped her relax and release the tensions of the day. When her work life became complicated and frustrating, she immediately thought of running as one of the ways to handle the stress that she felt. As a "Type A" kind of person, she enjoyed the multipurpose functions that running served for her.

EXERCISE: GOAL REFLECTION

Consider what your goals were at the beginning of your exercise journey and how they may have changed. Fill in the spaces below.

"When I first began exercising, my goals related to _____."

"Now that I've been exercising for _____, the following goals are the same:_____

_____

but these are different: _____."

Pattern Shifts and Boredom: Lapse and Relapse

"No matter what we do, the majority of people will relapse after any single attempt to overcome most chronic behavior problems" (Prochaska and Marcus 1994, p. 168). As I mentioned, approximately 50 percent of people embarking on exercise programs do not continue them more than six months. People cycle through the stages of change many times before finally ceasing undesired behaviors. Similarly, positive lifestyle changes may need to be tried a number of times before becoming permanent.

Relapse, or returning to your previous behavior, typically occurs when there are fluctuations in the routine or pattern of your life. In general, we can predict those types of situations likely to result in a shift back to the more familiar. These include: social pressures; changes in routine, whether that involves others' changes or your own (such as going on vacation); internal challenges; changes in weather; and illness or injury.

EXERCISE: PATTERN SHIFTS

Here are some common examples of pattern shifts. How might you handle them?

Your partner gives lip service to your physical activity but then somehow manages to ask you to watch the kids just at the moment that you're about to exercise.

I would: _____

_____

Special situations are ones that throw off any new behavior. Just as you're getting into a rhythm of exercise, you go on a vacation. You're in unfamiliar surroundings, and your daily pattern is different. How do you exercise then?

I would: _____

_____

Once you're back home, what will help you pick up where you left off?

I would: _____

_____

A family member becomes ill, and the spare time you had carved out for exercise disappears—and then time goes by.

I would: _____

_____

You have been exercising outdoors in the summer. Will you have the same flexibility come winter?

I would: _____

_____

You're drained of energy due to a cold, and so you stopped exercising. How do you get going again?

I would: _____

_____

List other possible patterns shifts in your life. What would you do to get going again?

_____

_____

_____

_____

_____

_____

- -

Internal challenges reflect those aspects of ourselves that really are much more comfortable with things the way they were—even if it didn't work very well, and even if we've moved beyond that particular understanding of ourselves. We all have what I think of as our "devil voice," that facet of our thinking that expresses contempt for what we are doing and asserts many reasons not to do it. This "voice" can in turn be successfully confronted by your "Silver Lining Voice," the part of you that really knows, appreciates, and understands the positive aspects of what is occurring.

■ Delia's Story

Delia thinks of herself as having a poor internal compass. When she goes to a strange city, she often gets lost, so she has tended to stay indoors. But since she started walking regularly, she has developed a new attitude about herself and her ability to navigate on her own. Now she finds herself eager to explore her environment on her daily two-mile walk. When she travels, she makes sure to get very clear written directions and take along a map of the town before she ventures outside. Along with these practical steps, she reminds herself how much she enjoys the freedom and flexibility of her new walking self. She is beginning to see herself in a different light, as someone who understands space as long as she uses the tools she's got and practices deliberately.

In order to maintain new exercise behaviors, it's especially important to find supports for your positive beliefs. Avoiding overconfidence is also critical. The old saying, "Pride goeth before the fall," is especially relevant in behavior change. Overconfidence can be a way to "court" relapse, since it involves a lack of mindfulness to important supports and warning signs and an over-reliance on your willpower to sustain change.

A variation on overconfidence is making small, seemingly irrelevant decisions that shift you back into old ways of behaving. Alan Marlatt, a psychologist at the University of Washington, specializes in issues of relapse and harm reduction. He refers to these decisions with the acronym "SUBTLE," that is: Seemingly Unimportant Behaviors That Lead to Errors.

At age fifty-three, Maria has caught on to some of her SUBTLE behaviors:

■ Maria's Story

Maria has recently begun swimming at the local hotel's pool. She's started and stopped swimming more times than she cares to count. And she knows herself well enough to predict that small obstacles are likely to derail her once more. One particular morning she was nearly at the pool when she realized that, though she had been clever enough to have dressed with her bathing suit under her clothes, she had forgotten to bring along underwear for after the swim. She sat in the hotel parking lot for a moment, trying to decide what to do with the limited time she had available before she had to be at work: skip the swim, drive back home and get dressed properly; no time to swim the rest of the week, there went her latest plans . . . Or . . .

The desk clerk let Maria use a hotel phone to call home. Her husband hadn't left for work yet, and he was going to drive by the hotel anyway. And yes, he was willing to stop by with her underwear in a plastic bag.

Although we may be completely motivated and although we may stay as conscious of our behavior as possible, we all are subject to minor disruptions of our intended activities. Being aware of our true intentions and being creative in solving minor problems can keep SUBTLEs from interfering in our lives.

Anticipating, predicting, and developing strategies for handling "lapses" helps keep them from becoming total relapses. It may not be possible to prevent relapse entirely, but the *degree* of backsliding can be addressed. In itself, a lapse isn't a problem. The problem arises when what we think and say to ourselves causes a lapse to lead rapidly to a relapse. Think of the dieter who has one bite of chocolate cake and concludes, "It's all over now." Or the person who has stopped drinking and figures "just one" won't hurt—and proceeds to get smashed, later feeling too ashamed to return to AA. These people are dealing with the "abstinence violation effect," our belief that one slip means that we have failed completely.

This same pattern of belief and behavior can happen, with the same emotional and cognitive reactions, when you lapse from positive changes. If you don't exercise when you intended to, does it become the occasion for discontinuing exercise? We might think of lapsing from a positive intention as a "health-habit violation effect"—the immediate dismantling of your entire exercise plan based on one instance of acting in a way other than you had planned. How you handle lapses, and whether you can keep lapses from becoming more extensive relapses, depends on what you say to yourself about yourself and what you believe about yourself.

One of the best methods of relapse prevention is relapse prediction. Many people, in fact, stop and resume exercising a number of times before developing a regular pattern of exercise. You can make use of this information about your own behavior to assist in your own planning, understanding more about yourself and the process of change.

EXERCISE: EXERCISE LAPSES AND RELAPSES

Based on what you know of yourself and your past exercise behavior, what would you predict could cause you to relapse? Here are some questions to get you started. Your responses to these questions give you the opportunity to think ahead, take responsibility for your exercising, and understand some of the motivational forces that are central to your exercising.

What might be high-risk situations for you?

_____

_____

What situations might get you off track?

_____

_____

What might be some "trigger events," that is, stressful thoughts or situations that might precede a relapse?

_____

_____

Are there some SUBTLEs that typically precede an exercise lapse for you?

_____

_____

How long would a lapse or relapse last?

_____

_____

How could you help yourself stay calm and rational?

_____

_____

What would help get you started again?

_____

_____

What would you need to do to renew your commitment to exercise?

_____

_____

How might you involve other people in helping you to get started again?

_____

_____

- -

If change is one predictor of relapse, the other major predictor is sameness—that is, boredom. What might be the predictors of boredom for you? A number of people get bored—and stop exercising—because of a sense of monotony, fixation on constant improvement, and/or a lack of company and an inward, negative focus. To counteract these potential problems, Dr. Joan Ullyot suggests varying your routine and exercising with friends whenever possible. "Talk, smell the flowers, enjoy the weather. And don't run so fast that all you can think about is getting enough air into your lungs and keeping your aching legs moving" (Ullyot 1976, pp. 16-17).

A sense of stagnation can become an opportunity to reevaluate your current reasons for exercising. These reasons may differ from those that got you started exercising. You might even want to develop a new Cost-Benefit Analysis for yourself, as you did in chapter 3. A typical challenge is the one faced by Conrad:

■ Conrad's Story

When I first began talking with forty-five-year-old Conrad, he reported a period of a few months during which he had bicycled regularly and enjoyed it immensely. A leg injury brought the biking to a halt. He was feeling extremely discouraged by a ride he'd had a few days before I talked with him: he found he could only ride a block before he became winded and his legs began to ache. He seemed to be waiting until, in some magical way, he would be transported back to his pre-injury self. Instead, I encouraged him to resume riding at the level at which his body was currently functioning and increase the distance only very gradually.

Sometimes it is useful to start with a clean slate, reassessing your priorities entirely. Although it may seem difficult to accept, relapse can become an opportunity for new understanding and change. My client Janice paused, regrouped, and started anew.

■ Janice's Story

Janice, a thirty-seven year-old professional with three young children, sought therapy because she was feeling overwhelmed and recognized that she wasn't taking care of herself adequately. A highly responsible person, she knew that she felt better when she took proper care of herself, yet some days she wouldn't brush her teeth, shower—or exercise. "I sabotage myself," she admitted. Feeling guilty, she dug her own hole deeper by lying to her husband, an avid exerciser. She would regularly tell him she had exercised when she hadn't.

The more Janice described her life stresses, the demands she placed on herself, and her distress and guilt, the more assured I felt in reversing my more typical recommendation. I encouraged her to give herself time off from exercise. Her immediate response was a feeling of great relief.

At the next session, we discussed how to contain this time off. Janice had described an "all or nothing" style in which she would make a strong commitment and then drop out of activities, giving up on herself. Even though she'd initially felt relieved not to *have* to exercise, she worried that this time off might really just be a new version of giving up on herself again. I suggested that she set a date by which she would review her decision. In this way, she would not feel a free-floating anxiety about exercise that would then result in new guilt and paralysis. Immediately she picked a date three weeks hence. She also decided to claim a personal "retreat" day to reflect: during half of the day she would review her personal life plans, and during the other half, the work decisions she needed to make.

Following that retreat week, Janice reported that she had specifically not exercised for two weeks. She now was starting to rebuild from the ground up. She and her husband were incorporating a regular weekly ski time together. She had decided to reestablish an enjoyable indoor tennis time with a friend. And then she could just decide to do some form of exercise on the weekends. Her husband, she recognized, used some of his weekend time in this way and would certainly support her in such a plan.

CHAPTER 10

"BUT IT FELT SO GOOD!": OVERDOING EXERCISE

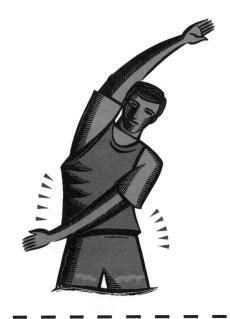

Up until now, we've been considering the positive and healthy aspects of exercising. But of course there also can be down sides. In this chapter, we'll consider the various ways in which exercise can get overused or misused. We'll look at exercise overuse in general. We'll also examine some particular instances in which overusing exercise can be a specific symptom of larger problems, such as among some people with eating disorders.

For the nonathlete, everyday exerciser, the likelihood of overuse is fairly slight. It reminds me of the proverbial newspaper headline: "Man bites dog." It might happen, but it's unlikely—and there's considerably more potential for the reverse. It's been estimated that less than 1 percent of the American population is at risk of overexercise.

I find that this topic comes up most frequently among people who point to incidents of overuse to justify their own inaction and lack of exercising at all. Exercise overuse becomes fodder for the "pre-contemplators" among us. It is *much* more likely that people will underuse rather than overuse exercise.

Nonetheless, do people who exercise sometimes get weird about their exercise? Yes! Is that weirdness sometimes a result of a variety of factors? Of course. Depending on the particular person, exercising too much may involve some combination of the following: inappropriate goals, a belief in your invincibility (or perhaps fears that are fueled by recognizing that you are merely mortal), drivenness, compensation, displacement, stress management, going into physiological "overdrive," as well as a response to others' demands or expectations.

As Dave Barry would say, this is a true story:

For some years, I have been a member of the "Psyching Team" at the New York City Marathon. Team members, who are mental health professionals and sport psychologists, chat with runners who have been bused out to Fort Wadsworth on Staten Island where the race takes place. We offer brief mental skills training interventions as the runners wait around before the race starts.

A few years ago, a worried-looking man approached me and asked whether I thought he should run. On the previous day, he explained, he was given an EKG (a measure of heart functioning). His physician told him the results were uncertain and expressed some concern about his running the marathon. Though he hadn't said anything directly to the runner, the physician had mentioned Jim Fixx to the man's wife. (Jim Fixx was a runner and popularizer of running who died of a heart attack—while running.)

I asked the man some questions about his health and risk factors. He appeared immovably indecisive. Finally, concerned that I was getting nowhere and that I might be dealing with a medical rather than a psychological issue, I introduced the runner to Harold Selman, M.D., the psychiatrist who co-leads the Psyching Team. Dr. Selman asked similar questions and received correspondingly inconclusive replies. Dr. Selman assured the man a place in the race the following year if he decided not to run this year. Still, nothing seemed settled. Finally Dr. Selman pulled out the big card: "Which is more important," he asked, "your life or this race?" At this, the man suddenly drew himself up, all doubt resolved. With conviction he stated, "I'll run."

The next day I carefully checked the *New York Times*. There were no reports of death on the race course.

Moderation in All Things: The Psychophysiological and Psychosocial Costs of Overuse

People don't usually set out to exercise too much, but sometimes the behavior takes over. Overuse can occur among "weekend warriors," committed exercisers, collegiate athletes, and professional athletes. There are a number of costs—to the mind as well as the body.

In our quintessentially American faith that more is better, we sometimes become caught in a dangerous trap. As we've reviewed here, we know that exercise in moderation can lead to improved self-concept, mastery, self-efficacy, self-sufficiency, body image, and cognitive processing. But too much exercise can result in negative effects. Sometimes people overtrain in order to meet performance goals (Raglin 1993) or in an attempt to control weight—or life—through compulsive or obligatory exercise (Yates 1991). People who exercise more than their bodies can tolerate and leave too little time for restorative recovery are at increased risk of sustaining specific as well as training-stress injuries. The Greek aphorism "Moderation in all things" is an important exercise rule to follow.

A number of physiological signs can tell you when you're doing too much. These might include sleep disturbance, increased illness and injury, chronic muscle soreness, and elevated resting heart rate and blood pressure. But the psychosocial symptoms may be even more apparent—and paradoxical. These are the opposite of the beneficial aspects of exercise. Too much exercise can leave people with fatigue, problems with concentration, apathy, anger, irritability, depression, and impaired social relations. Sport performance deteriorates. Athletes sometimes compound the problem by increasing their training in a futile attempt to improve their performance (Henschen 1993; McCann 1995; Raglin 1993).

Usually when we think about something as being objectively and actually true, we look to the physical realm. We tend to think that our thoughts or feelings might be more subjective—and subject to our own interpretations. Interestingly, when it comes to signs of exercise overuse, various studies have suggested that even with various fine-tuned physiological measurement, the *psychological* signs are often more accurate predictors of exercise overuse than are the physiological indicators (Morgan et al. 1988; Theriault, Richard, Labrie, and Theriault 1997).

How much exercise is too much? We have no exact measures. "Too much" depends to some extent on the individual—your personality, your lifestyle, your level of training, and the circumstances in which you exercise. If you've been exercising over a period of time and have experienced the mental and physical benefits of exercise but are now showing some of the physical or mental signs of overuse, that may be a signal for you to review and reflect on whether you're overusing exercise. It may be that you've markedly increased any of the FIT variables of exercise. Or you may be experiencing other kinds of stressors and your body is signaling "Something's gotta give." If exercise that was fun and interesting now seems obligatory and you are in a constant state of energy depletion, sort of like chronic jet lag, this may be another sign. Your family and friends may be concerned that you're doing too much. But you need to pay attention to the source. Do these people understand what you're doing and why? Are they people who don't exercise and may be a bit overprotective? Or are you rationalizing for yourself behavior that really *isn't* healthy for you? This is another of those moments when you may need to take a fearless inventory: pay attention to your particular situation and your specific mental and physical reactions.

EXERCISE: ARE YOU OVERDOING IT?

There is no absolute measure of exercise overuse. However, here are some key questions you can ask yourself:

PHYSIOLOGICAL AND PSYCHOLOGICAL SIGNS

Have any of the following been present for me on a routine basis recently (*not* due to medical condition, psychological condition, or changed life circumstances):

Physiological

_____ Elevated morning resting pulse rate

_____ Increase in injuries

_____ Chronic muscle soreness

_____ Frequent minor infections

_____ Decreased appetite or weight loss

Psychological

_____ Fatigue

_____ Reduced concentration

_____ Irritability

_____ Depression

_____ Insomnia

SOCIAL AND BEHAVIORAL SIGNS

_____ When I'm sick or injured, am I able to decrease or stop exercising long enough to recover?

_____ If I miss an exercise session, do I feel anxious or uncomfortable?

_____ Do I use exercise as self-punishment?

_____ Do I neglect business, family, or social responsibilities because of my exercise schedule?

_____ Do I continually try to exercise more or harder?

If I had a best friend who exercised in the way I do, what would I say to him or her about whether they were overusing exercise?

_____

_____

_____

What advice would I give my friend if I thought they were doing too much?

_____

_____

- -

What's in a Name?

The overuse of exercise goes by a number of names. Within sport psychology circles, there are arguments about whether to call it staleness or burnout, overtraining or negative stress response. More popularly, people sometimes describe this problem as "exercise addiction" or "compulsive exercise." Some research would seem to support this latter perspective. When committed runners followed an experimental plan to *not* exercise, their moods deteriorated (Mondin et al. 1996). This decrease in mood when exercise is withheld could be interpreted to mean that exercise is addictive and that they were suffering "withdrawal" symptoms. But if we use the perspective that exercise is natural, then lack of exercise would feel uncomfortable. Using our early comparison with sleep once again: if we don't get sleep for a night, would we describe the resulting feelings a function of "sleep addiction" or ourselves as "compulsive sleep seekers"? These terms imply some things about motivation and causation. If you're highly motivated, does that mean that you have an "addictive" or "compulsive" personality? Since that's not always either descriptively or diagnostically accurate, I will stay with the more neutral term, "overuse."

To understand how and why exercise overuse can happen, let me tell you about one of my clients:

■ George's Story

George, a thirty-year-old triathlete, was referred to me by his orthopedic surgeon. He was experiencing tendinitis, an inflammation of the tendons in his legs. The orthopedist had recommended a four- to six-week moratorium on exercise to resolve the problem. George, however, found even the *idea* of this length of time without exercise intolerable. He had tried an occasional day off from working out, but as soon as his pain eased up, he resumed his routine. And the tendinitis wasn't healing.

George said that he was feeling short-tempered, overwhelmed at work, gloomy, tired, and without energy. A gangly, adolescent-looking man, George was emotionally immature as well. He had few friends, no history of dating, and a highly stressful and unsatisfying job. Triathlon competitions provided a major focus for his life and structure for his self-definition.

George recognized that his physician's recommendation made sense. And yet the thought of even a week's respite was unimaginable to him. We talked about what it was that was preventing George from resting—and also some ways he could challenge these beliefs. For example, he worried about losing conditioning if he didn't run for a day or two. He recognized, though, that he could remind himself: "I'll maintain enough, and it would come back, especially if I continue with swimming and Nautilus." Whereas his first thought was, "If I don't do this physical activity or compete, it feels like someone's pulled my legs out from under me," he acknowledged that he needed to pay attention to other sources of self-esteem. He had been labeling himself a "failure," but he understood that "Other athletes have to take time off, too—and they don't like it either."

George's family background provided the emotional starting point of his current dilemma. He had grown up the only child of an alcoholic mother and a physically abusive stepfather. Like many children of abusive and dysfunctional households, he had hoped and acted as if his behavior would change his parents' behavior. He was studious and cooperative; as often and for as long as possible, he spent time outside his house and away from the conflict there. He wandered outside for hours, dreading the return home. For him, there was a direct connection between the relief from emotional tension and being physically active outside.

As he understood more about his lifelong and characteristic approach to stress, George began changing his work and social life. He developed some close friendships through attending a group for adult children of alcoholics. He started to broaden his interests and activities. He examined his triathlon training and racing. By simultaneously graphing his level of training, his triathlon results, and his work stress, he could see some patterns: More training did not necessarily result in improved race performance. Further, his always-stressful job became seasonally more challenging exactly at peak racing time.

This graph proved a turning point for George's life planning: he began designing a more reasonable and pleasurable approach to the next racing season, choosing two-event, rather than three-event, races. Despite some job adjustments, he recognized that he was chronically unhappy in that work setting. Ultimately, he quit that job, opting to try his hand at work he enjoyed.

George was never able to stop exercising completely, but he did tolerate two weeks without running or bicycling—while continuing to swim the entire time. The tendinitis healed, and his mood improved. In the process, George learned to be more systematic in his training. He built in nonworkout days and learned not to be scared of sitting still.

EXERCISE: AUTOMATIC THOUGHTS AND RATIONAL RESPONSES

If, like George, you are overusing exercise, what basic assumptions and beliefs prevent you from pausing long enough to let your body recover? Write down those assumptions or "automatic thoughts." Next to them, counter those concerns and beliefs with rational commentary.

Automatic Thought Regarding Exercise	*Rational Response Regarding Exercise*
EXAMPLE:	
If I don't exercise today, I will gain two pounds.	It takes more than one missed exercise session to gain that much weight. Besides, my body is telling me that exercising today will mean that I'll have a cold tomorrow.
1. _____ _____	_____ _____
2. _____ _____	_____ _____
3. _____ _____	_____ _____

General Recommendations for Handling Exercise Overuse

At what point does athletic training move from pressured to taxing? When does exercise shift from enjoyable to driven? While there are no absolute rules—the point of shift may well be internally consistent for any one person. This "slippery slope" involves a combination of your exercise history, current physiological demand, and other psychosocial pressures and stressors.

Two elements are critical in learning to handle exercise overuse: learning not only the "what" but also the "why." When you ask yourself these difficult but important questions, you give yourself the opportunity to learn much from your responses to yourself. My friend Stephanie, now thirty-two, learned a few years ago not only the "why"s but the "what to do about it"s, as well.

■ Stephanie's Story

For five years, Stephanie had biked fiercely. She used the intensity of her exercise to avoid experiencing negative emotions. She called these her "angry, scary, sad feelings. I biked to such an extreme that I ended up with an injured body. I was always riding more, faster. Bigger gears, steeper hills. I was exercising while angry, hurt, and tense—and not even realizing it. All that tension and the big gears and the hills—bad combo. I ended up with some serious disk problems. It forced me off my bike and onto my feet. I always thought not biking would kill me, that I would instantly become fat, unhappy, and unlovable."

Stephanie had to retrain her brain and her body as well as revise her exercise program. She learned to feel her emotions in the moment. "Somehow, knowing that when I don't really express my emotions, I'll feel it in my back instead scared me into really wanting to change."

Over time, Stephanie learned to adjust her exercise and try different types of exercise that she now loves. "At first I couldn't accept anything else as 'real' exercise. Walking felt wimpy at first. Then I got into swimming. And hiking. Yoga. Even returned to some biking. Exercise was a bit transformed for me. I didn't perform it to quite the extreme point I had in the past. It's not that I don't have these tendencies anymore—I still do. But I can enjoy the activity for what it is."

Stephanie turned the experience of overusing exercise into an opportunity to learn about the body-mind relationship. "It taught me so much about myself. It forced me to look at what I was doing to myself physically and psychologically. I realized I was beating myself up in my head, always thinking I should do more, because I was channeling my entire emotional self into my bike riding. I learned to be more assertive in real life, not just ultra-aggressive on my bike. I learned how to feel my feelings, not bury them and save them for a ride. I still use exercise as a way to help me process my emotions, but that's different from swapping a hard physical workout for feeling emotions."

If you can learn to recognize your own "warning signs," ultimately you will be able to develop a sense of control of your exercise, rather than having it control you. Although there aren't any right or wrong answers, your reactions can help you understand more about yourself and your own patterns of thought, feeling, and behavior.

JOURNAL TASK: REFLECTIONS ON OVERUSE

In addition to the reflective exercise, "Are You Overdoing It?" above, you can use your journal to consider this topic from a number of angles.

1. *Warning Signs:* You can ask yourself questions such as:
   What are the physical signals that tell me that I'm pushing my exercise too hard?
   What are the mental signals that tell me that I'm pushing my exercise too hard?
   What purpose does exercise serve in my life?
   What is it I'm avoiding?
   What changes do I want to make?

2. *Tracking Overuse:* In your logbook or journal, develop a method for tracking and ultimately predicting periods of high training stress. This can be a chart with checkmarks or symbols to indicate the physiological and psychological signs of overuse. It can also have a more reflective bent, in which you examine in depth some of the issues of control, safety, body image, or identity that seem to form the basis of your tendency toward exercise overuse.

A number of practical strategies can either help you slow down the development of exercise overuse or recover once you're in the midst of it.

Just Say No

Intentionally schedule some "off-periods" during which you don't exercise at all. But please note: If you are an avid exerciser like George, vacations from exercise may feel extremely difficult, especially at first. You may need to apply the sense of discipline that you usually use for the purpose of getting you out and exercising for *not* exercising in order to allow your body to rest. You might also specifically plan other things to do, as a way of distracting yourself from your tendency to exercise. Or you might want to plan a specific "reward" you'll give yourself for this time-out.

Cross-Training

Cross-training (involving other sports that use different muscles) can be helpful, and can often serve as a preventative of further structural problems. For example, weight training might become a substitute for running a few days per week, thus increasing your upper body strength while giving your legs a rest. (Your running stamina is likely to improve through this cross-training.)

Picture This

Mental practice periods, in which you use mental imagery of your sport, can serve to break up the monotony of practice, allow your body to recuperate physically, and help you recognize the power of imagery.

Stay Sociable

If part of the value of exercise for you includes the opportunity to spend time with others, you can engage in noncompetitive, nonstressful social team activities. These can enhance your sense of peer connection without bodily strain.

Stay Competitive—If You Wish

If part of the pleasure of exercise for you involves competition, you might participate in other types of competitive activities so that you can maintain your "fighting edge" without compromising your body.

An Ounce of Prevention

If you're involved in competitive sports, learning how to handle postcompetition tension can serve a preventative function, since some postcompetition reactions may relate to training stress.

Who's Controlling What?

At a more psychological level, it's useful to remember that one of the emotional dynamics of overuse is the attempt to maintain control. Perhaps other aspects of your life feel out of control. Examining those issues and concerns directly allows you to begin to address rather than avoid them. If you feel that you are not in control of your training schedule, there may be some ways in which you can increase the choices and options available to you—thus increasing your sense of control.

- -

EXERCISE: STRATEGIES

To which of the above strategies do you want to commit yourself? Check off the ones that apply. Record what you *actually* do, so that you can assess its effectiveness in decreasing the likelihood of overuse or assisting in your recovery:

1. "Exercise-free" zones

2. Cross-training

3. Mental practice

4. Noncompetitive social team activities

5. Nonexercise competitive activities

6. Predicting and managing postcompetition reactions

7. Attention to issues of control

- -

Moving now from general issues of exercise overuse, let's look at the ways in which exercise is sometimes *mis*used through overuse as a method of weight control and weight management.

Bulimia: The Vicious Cycle

Many aspects of our well-being are related to balance and self-regulation. At its simplest, our patterns of eating reflect that balance. All other things being equal, if you eat and exercise normally, you will maintain or lose weight. If you persistently overeat or binge eat, you will gain weight.

But our natural bodily patterns and rhythms of eating can become disregulated in a variety of ways. Some are cyclical and set into action a perpetual motion machine. Bulimia is one of those. The sequence of binging and restriction typically involves a cycle of food restriction, followed by extreme hunger with consequent overeating, with resulting guilt and shame, in turn leading to efforts to rid yourself of the effects of the action. Subsequent restriction maintains the vicious cycle. Most commonly, people use vomiting or laxatives as methods of purging. A number of people use high-intensity aerobic exercise for a sort of self-punishing weight control.

We all overeat some of the time or eat when we are not especially hungry. And many people are motivated to exercise in part for weight control. Likewise, there are many social supports for being thin and for exercise (Rodin 1992). The issue of bulimic exercise, then, is more a matter of degree than kind. It's really a combination of intention and emotion (Walsh and Garner 1997).

Some of this is also related to gender. The eating disorders of restriction, bulimia and anorexia, are largely gender-specific disorders. These disorders may represent the extreme version of women's "typical" concerns around weight (Rodin, Silberstein, and Striegel-Moore 1984). My client Erica illustrates these issues.

■ Erica's Story

A long and lanky twenty-nine-year-old, Erica had a fifteen-year history of disregulated eating. She had been anorexic and now was bulimic. Erica tackled exercise as she did everything else: chaotically and with a vengeance. She performed running and aerobics with determination but without a plan. Excesses followed droughts. Driving herself physically was gratifying to this woman who felt little satisfaction with most of her life. Exercise was yet another venue to punish herself while ostensibly doing the "right thing."

As she developed greater self-acceptance, Erica also gradually let go of binging and purging. Exercise, too, took on a predictable pattern, one that allowed her to experience pleasure in activity for its own sake.

The reality of bulimia can be physically damaging and is experienced as extremely distressing and out of control. The distinguishing characteristic of bulimic exercise is that, rather than perceiving exercise as energizing and pleasurable, exercise is meted out in a desperate attempt to right the scales. Obligatory intensity diminishes the possible psychological benefits. You may have begun exercise to balance out overeating yet found yourself caught in a cycle in which one action seems to justify and necessitate its opposite reaction. The negative consequences can be physically and psychologically damaging.

Exercise Recommendations for People with Bulimia

As with other forms of purging, if you are bulimic and use exercise as a self-perpetuating attempt at balancing or undoing the effects of binges, the most important thing that you can do is learn how to figuratively or even literally "stand still." This may be something that you can do on your own, or it may be important to work with a therapist who can help you figure out ways to feel emotionally safe while doing this important and difficult work.

JOURNAL TASKS: PATTERN EXAMINATION

Even though there aren't accurate measures to determine excessive exercise, you can begin looking at your patterns of thoughts and actions in relation to food, eating, exercise, guilt, and self-punishment.

1. You can write freely on these topics.

2. You can develop a chart to track your eating and exercise patterns. Adapting a monitoring record developed by Fairburn (1995), your chart would look like the one on the next page.

3. Develop a chart in which you keep track of your automatic thoughts and rational responses regarding eating and exercise.

4. A journal "dialogue" between yourself and exercise can assist you in understanding the role of exercise in perpetuating your bulimic behavior. As the internal "battle" involving binging, punishment, and deprivation becomes more visible and obvious to you, you will feel more control over ways you can intervene in your own behavior. By clarifying, recognizing, and naming your concerns, you can address and resolve them.

As with other disorders of eating, the ultimate goal is for you to regain a sense of food as food, weight as only one aspect of your self-definition, eating as related to actual physiological hunger, and exercise as part of connecting with your entire (including bodily) self.

Monitoring Record

Day _____   Date _____

Time	Food/drink consumed	Situation	*	V/L/E	Context and comments

Explanation of columns:

Keep track of time of day and record everything you eat or drink, including binge items. Write down the information as soon as possible after eating.

Situation: Note the situation of your eating, such as where you were and whether alone or with other(s)

*: Put an asterisk (*) in this column if you felt that any of the food items were excessive. A binge would be indicated by a cluster of asterisks.

V/L/E: If you used some method of purging, such as vomiting (V), laxatives (L), or excessive exercise (E), note that in this column.

Add any feelings or descriptive or explanatory comments in the final column.

Anorexia and Ascetic Exercise

Bulimia is designed as a balancing act. In contrast, the drive toward power via nothingness forms the seductive core of anorexia. Anorexia has been described as the "relentless pursuit of thinness" (Bruch 1978). Experienced as a companion, a means, and/or a slave master, exercise can be swept up in that relentless pursuit. To be able to run endless hours signals the triumph of will over body. If you use excessive exercise as part of your anorexic pattern, recovery may be especially challenging for you (Casper and Jabine 1996). My client Diana experienced this dilemma:

◼ Diana's Story

An exquisite, stylishly dressed, petite young woman with flowing blond hair, thirty-year-old Diana came to therapy because she realized that her food preoccupation and exercise for weight control had almost entirely shut out her social life. "My whole life is targeted on diet and exercise," she commented. After a full day of work, she regularly rode her exercise bicycle for three hours, ending up exhausted and drained. She had neither energy nor time for her new marriage. She did not allow space or time for the development of friendships or other activities.

Diana described a history of disordered eating and weight control for at least the past eleven years. She had used laxatives and vomiting for weight control, and starved herself, sometimes for days. When I first saw her, she was subsisting on little food and lots of exercise. She recognized that she was trying to control both anxiety and depression through her weight preoccupation. She felt caught in the cycle, out of control of her rumination and behavior. She knew her marriage was in trouble. She had attended couples therapy briefly—but dropped out because it interfered with her workouts.

Initially eager to attend a therapy group for women with bulimia and/or anorexia, Diana responded to the group by feeling competitive and increasing her exercise. Individual therapy, psychotropic medication, and, gradually, community support allowed her to begin developing alternate ways for feeling some level of safety and control in the world.

Our bodies and minds—our beings—are designed so that, below a certain body weight, our thinking becomes much less rational and reasonable. One of the indicators of anorexia nervosa is that a person's body weight is at least 15 percent below their ideal body weight. This was part of the challenge of working with Diana—she literally needed to weigh more in order to have enough brain fuel to think more clearly about her problems and their solution.

When I work with people who have an anorexic style and anorexic beliefs, but weigh "merely" 10 percent rather than 15 percent below their ideal body weight, we can often make much better progress:

◼ Martha's Story

Martha was also thirty, an academic researcher with a childlike voice to match her perky, adolescent looks. Since college, she had severely restricted her eating. She also exercised daily, vigorously, for a few hours each time. At five-foot-four, she maintained her weight around 100 pounds. She described herself as always tired, not especially happy, perfectionistic, and continuously preoccupied with thoughts of food.

Martha was surprised and doubtful but intrigued at the idea that eating more and eating in more varied fashion could actually mean that she wouldn't be thinking about food all the time. We examined her list of "food rules" and sorted the list into three categories: appropriate and healthy; rules that make sense for people who need to lose weight; and "MWI"—Martha's Wacky Ideas; that is, food restrictions that she had developed that only served to limit her—and were often impossible to meet. For example, Martha was conscious of the fat levels of various dairy products such as sour cream, cream cheese, mayonnaise, and cheese. She limited dairy to nonfat milk and yogurt. Although she was inhibiting some food choices, there was underlying rationality to this decision, both in terms of health and potential for weight loss. On the other hand, one of her rules was "Put off meals for as long as possible. Go to bed early to avoid dinner." This prohibition was based entirely on a battle of wills between Martha and her body. It bore no relationship to any aspect of health.

As we continued to explore Martha's unrealistic expectations of herself, she also began working with a nutritionist. Gradually, she broadened out the numbers and kinds of food that she would eat. She became generally more self-accepting. Martha was willing to be persuaded that working out only four days a week would allow a better balance in her life. She gained a few pounds and was excited to find that life in general was more fun and that she had more energy. Her research work felt more interesting and engaging. She was startled and delighted to realize that she wasn't thinking about food all the time. She continued to miss her period—regular menstruation often disappears when women drop below a body weight sufficient to support a healthy pregnancy—but she remained unconvinced that this was her body's way of telling her that she was still underweight.

EXERCISE: My Food Rules

1. Like Martha, you can write down all the "rules" that you maintain about yourself and food, weight and eating.

2. Categorize these rules as
   - **H**—Rules that make sense for any person who wants to eat healthily
   - **WL**—Rules that make sense for a person who needs to lose weight
   - **I**—Idiosyncratic rules that you've developed for yourself (probably involving restriction)

3. Once you have written out all your rules and categorized them, rewrite a reasonable or healthy list for yourself. This list can be described as "principles" or "guidelines" rather than "rules."

Caution: If you have an eating disorder, it may be very difficult for you to maintain objectivity about your situation and your assumptions about yourself. This exercise may work best if reviewed with somebody else, whether a therapist or a close (but objective) friend.

Over the past ten years, a number of researchers have addressed the connection between eating disorders and exercise, attempting to understand whether there is a cause and effect relationship. One line of thought compares anorexia to the asceticism of medieval saints and martyrs (Bordo 1993; Yates 1991). This austerity focuses on purification, will, discipline, the conquest of desire, aspiration toward an ideal, and transcendence of the body. Extremes of exercise can fit naturally into this pattern. Whether it is causally connected or coincidental, both committed exercisers and people with anorexia tend to be perfectionistic, achievement oriented, highly motivated, able to tolerate physical discomfort, and approval-seeking (Thompson and Sherman 1993). But the fine line between positive drive and preoccupied drivenness can sometimes be breached.

In a number of studies designed to tease out the interaction of eating disorders, obsessive characteristics, and exercise, Caroline Davis and her colleagues at York University in Toronto have compared anorexic inpatients with corresponding groups of community members, focusing in particular on the relative frequency and duration of exercise. They suggest that an interacting triad of related factors—exercise, obsessive compulsiveness, and dieting—appears to be the basis for eating disorders. "The relationships among physical activity, starvation, and obsessive compulsiveness tend to be reciprocal and dynamic" (Davis et al. 1995, p. 974), potentiating each other in a destructive, self-perpetuating loop.

Epling and Pierce (1991) have suggested that, rather than being a result of the drive for thinness, physical activity in and of itself can be associated with, cause, or exacerbate anorexia. They have termed this condition "activity anorexia," which they define as:

> the loss of appetite that occurs when physical activity interferes with eating....
> The first effect of combining dieting and exercise is that physical activity accelerates to excessive levels. As exercise increases, the value of food declines and people eat less. Paradoxically, as food intake decreases (i.e. deprivation) the motivation to exercise increases. (Epling and Pierce, 1991, p. 111)

In a paradoxical manner, they suggest, food restriction increases physical activity, the activity affects physiological processes, and these in turn lead to increased food restriction. "Once initiated, this cycle of increasing activity and decreasing food intake is resistant to change" (Epling and Pierce 1991, p. 9).

Epling and Pierce propose that there may be physiological bases for this behavior. In evolutionary terms, like hungry rats learning the way through a maze to get to the food reward, activity as a response to starvation may have the functional value of increasing the likelihood of finding food. The endogenous (coming from inside us) opiates potentially produced by exercise, those brain chemicals that help us feel good, may decrease appetite. Because of cultural conditioning, women more than men are likely to use diet and exercise in such a way that the biobehavioral process of activity anorexia is initiated. "Activity anorexia is therefore a biobehavioral process activated by cultural requirements for thinness and fitness" (Epling and Pierce 1991, p. 168).

Recommendations for People with Anorexia

As with bulimia, when exercise takes on a different function and even becomes a symptom, it is important to discontinue its destructive use and begin moving toward healthy or at least moderated exercise. If you are anorexic and reading this book, it is my fervent hope (and plea) that this reading is serving as a supplement to some additional forms of treatment. Anorexia can rarely be resolved on its own.

A number of inpatient programs prohibit exercise among anorexic patients, but enforcement may be challenging. Sometimes the prohibition against exercise becomes a place for patients to do battle with staff. Unfortunately, all this means is that the central psychological issues about control are getting played out in yet another place and with new people. An alternative possibility is a supervised exercise program that can serve "the major goal of therapy—namely, to facilitate the patients' responsibility for themselves, rather than to increase feelings of helplessness, resentment, and dependence" (Beumont, Beumont, Touyz, and Williams 1997, p. 186).

When you can view physical activity as part of the re-connection between your self and your body, it can serve a therapeutic function. Yoga or walking can be especially helpful if there are physiological or compulsive aspects to your exercise. These forms of exercise may involve less energy expenditure. Equally significant, yoga and walking can also provide excellent opportunities for you to attend to yourself in the present moment.

Ultimately, changes in exercise patterns are a part of the overall change of focus you are developing about yourself and your body. Moving toward an appreciation of yourself as having value and worth in your own being, you can gradually attend more to those aspects of your life that will help you feel healthy. Exercise is one such component. Instead of exercise as self-flagellation, you will be able to begin to recognize or regain a sense of the pleasure inherent in movement. At least initially, however, you will need to continue to guard against old habits. You can make use of the seductive pull of overexercise as a cue to the ways in which your life may be feeling out of control. Symptom then becomes signal, allowing you opportunity for change.

CHAPTER 11

IS FOOD EATING YOU?

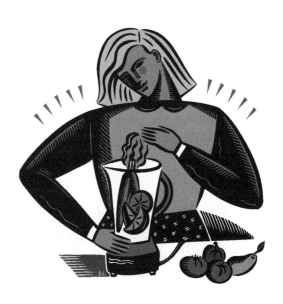

In the previous chapter, we saw how exercise can be used as a negative means of coping—a way of avoiding or escaping from concerns that need to be addressed directly. More typical than that scenario, however, is the use of food—or other substances—to cover over, mask, or avoid those same types of concerns. This chapter is designed to look at the ways in which exercise can be a constructive method for changing some of these other negative health habits. The most obvious is the unhealthy use of food, but later in the chapter, we'll also look at the relationship between alcohol and smoking cessation and exercise. As we saw before, when you exercise, you align yourself with healthy habits that in their own way assist you in becoming healthier all around.

Food, Weight, and Exercise

Exercise is connected with food and weight in a number of ways. It can help regulate appetite, alter food preferences, and reinforce healthier eating habits. Another part of the positive cycle is that, as you feel more confident about exercise, you may experience greater self-confidence and more positive thoughts and mood regarding weight management (Rodin 1992). Through exercise, your body shape begins to change so that you *appear* leaner, even if you stay at the same weight. My own experience taught me some unanticipated lessons about exercise, food, and appearance.

When I started running and discovered my passion for being physically active it did not occur to me that this behavior would have benefits other than feeling better physically. The first thing I noticed was that my thought processes changed (see chapter 8). I probably slept better—or at least, less badly, since this was a time of crisis in my life. What I didn't anticipate was that running would affect what I ate and how my body looked.

A few weeks after I had begun running, while thinking about what I would have for dinner, I decided, "I'd like some chicken tonight." I couldn't recall when I'd last eaten chicken. And then, in growing surprise, I wondered when I had last eaten beef, pork, or lamb. Fish? Without noticing, I had wiped out the major sources of protein in my diet. This hadn't been intentional—it had just happened as a result of my checking inside to see what my body hunger suggested. Outside of my awareness, I had become a vegetarian. My next step was learning about alternative sources of protein!

I've never become entirely a vegetarian, actually. I still occasionally do eat fish and fowl. But the very thought of the "pleasures" of eating red meat entirely disappeared from my consciousness—as an effect of running.

I also noticed that my clothes began to fit me differently. Though I did lose a few pounds, what most surprised me as someone naive to this effect was that my body took on a more defined and muscular shape. It seemed clear to me that this was how my body was "supposed" to look, now that I was taking proper care of it.

A Trip Down "Gender Lane": Gender, Weight, Diet, and Exercise

If we're going to talk about food and eating, we need to take a side trip along "gender lane." In our society, food, eating, weight, and exercise have gender-specific elements and meanings. Within our culture, it is typical for women to be preoccupied about food, weight, and body issues (Bordo 1993). "For an overwhelming number of women in our society, being a woman means feeling too fat" (Rodin, Silberstein, and Striegel-Moore 1984, p. 267).

Women's bodies have been turned into objects for centuries. "Women's bodies have always and everywhere been perceived as unfinished, in want of carving, perforating, incising, refining, and realignment" (Rodin, 1992, p. 24). Women's bodies become a "mobile billboard for their owner's brilliance, energy, and savvy" (p. 26).

Women bond and compete around issues of thinness and physical attractiveness. Focus on food and weight is a means of connection, sometimes through the media (such as women's magazines) or more personally (a friend's struggle with her latest diet). At the same time, these areas "may be the chief and most wholeheartedly sanctioned competitive domains in which women are encouraged to contend with each other" (Rodin, Silberstein, and Striegel-Moore 1984, p. 290).

Being sensitive to others' thoughts and feelings is one of the important aspects of growing up female in our culture. But there is a down side to this relational sensitivity. We women live life comparing ourselves to one another—and comparing ourselves internally to an airbrushed, unattainable, idealized, fantasy woman promoted by the media.

Additional gender differences occur in regard to weight preoccupation, weight loss, and maintenance of that loss. As if it were a diabolical plot, women are at a number of sociocultural and physiological disadvantages regarding an issue that tends to have much more meaning for us. In general, men are less encumbered by the sociocultural web surrounding the interaction of food, eating, nurturance, and weight. Men typically have more lean body mass and less body fat than women, and since lean tissue is more metabolically active than fat, tend to have a higher metabolic rate (Thompson and Sherman 1993). With higher resting metabolic rates, men require more calories to sustain general functioning. And since they have not dieted as frequently as women—women are twice as likely as men to report that they are dieting to lose weight (Stephenson, Levy, Sass, and McGarvey 1987)—men's bodies have not developed the metabolic slowdown that results from weight cycling (Rodin 1992; Striegel-Moore, Silberstein, and Rodin 1986). Thus, they tend to be able to lose weight and maintain weight loss more readily. And men more easily turn to exercise for weight control than do women.

Even though I have focused on women's issues in relation to weight, men do not escape our cultural preoccupation with how we look. Men certainly have concerns around weight, body image, self-esteem, and exercise. For example, a research study of overweight men participating in either weight reduction or aerobic conditioning found that their general mental health improved over time. In contrast, the control subjects (overweight men not participating in the program) showed an increase in levels of depression (Koeppl et al. 1992).

More Weight Equals Less Activity

Approximately thirty-four million adults in the U.S. are obese. Of those, twenty million are women. Another twenty million women are overweight or think that they are (Kirschenbaum 1992). Inactivity contributes more to the maintenance of obesity than does overeating (Heil and Henschen 1996). And there is the interaction of inactivity and obesity: "as weight increases activity decreases" (Heil and Henschen 1996, p. 241).

Why Exercise Works

Exercise and weight loss are associated in a number of ways. Most obvious is the sheer balancing act of caloric intake versus expenditure. Exercise uses up more calories than does sitting still. There are additional benefits as well. When you decreases caloric intake through dieting alone, your metabolism is suppressed, which actually slows down your body's functioning. In contrast, exercise serves to increase your body's resting metabolic rate. As an added bonus, your body continues at a higher metabolic rate for a time after exercise, thus maintaining more efficient functioning (and burning more fuel, that is, calories, in the process). Despite what people sometimes assume, moderate exercise actually tends to decrease rather than increase your appetite. As happened with me, exercise may also change your food preferences toward more balanced eating (Foreyt and Goodrick 1992; Grilo 1996). Since muscle burns more calories than does fat, increase in muscle mass (through exercise) results in greater caloric loss. In contrast to other methods of weight loss, exercise attacks body fat rather than lean body tissue. Exercise appears to be the one method for lowering your "set point," the balancing weight regulation mechanism that tends to keep people at a stable weight (Kirschenbaum 1994).

In addition to the physical effects, there are a number of positive psychological effects of exercise in relation to weight loss. Along with general improvements in mood associated with exercise, people often experience an increased feeling of control as well as a sense of self-efficacy. Some people have a sense that "if I can take charge of my exercising self, I can make choices about what and when I eat." Further, exercise may have a profound impact on both body awareness and hunger awareness (Sheehan 1978), each an important aspect of weight loss. Learning to take charge was important in my client Joyce's life:

■ Joyce's Story

Defiantly, forty-year-old Joyce exclaimed, "I don't want to diet anymore!" She was startled when I responded with equal intensity: "Great!" A much-silenced mother of three who worked in her husband's business, she had entered therapy with tearfulness, fatigue, low self-esteem, and fuming irritability. Being overweight added to her sense of shame and social isolation.

After we had discussed various options, Joyce decided to walk with her neighbor and their children to and from the school bus stop on a daily basis. Shortly after that, she told her (surprised) husband of her general wretched unhappiness. Talking with him then gave her the courage to talk with a friend and begin to feel less alone with her pain. She commented that this was the first time she had ever started to lose weight by developing a regular pattern of exercise prior to the initiation of dieting. Though she wished to lose weight, she was now really clear that she did not want to go on a diet.

We discussed the virtues of lifestyle and habit change rather than quick but backfiring "fixes." Joyce was intrigued by referral to a registered dietitian who conducted a group on healthy weight management. Empowered by her now-predictable walking pattern, she transferred that sense of self-efficacy to the potential for weight loss.

The satisfaction of movement can have metaphorical as well as transferred meaning. As you become accustomed to exercise, this activity can come to be experienced as a different way of "feeding" yourself, nourishing your body and clearing your mind.

Losing Weight

This book is not specifically about weight loss, so I will only make a few comments here having to do with your perspective on yourself and your weight. There are some things we know for sure. Fad diets (no matter how they are couched as the latest breakthrough amazing weight loss discovery) really do not work. To be effective, weight loss must be a gradual process and must involve changes in various lifestyle patterns.

What is the right weight for you? Probably not some unattainable "ideal" that was developed for actuarial charts. Much more significant is a healthy or reasonable weight. This number (or more likely, weight range) needs to take into account your family's weight history and patterns, your lowest weight for over a year as an adult, the largest size clothes you'd feel comfortable wearing, your perception of "normal" weight among your family or friends, and what weight you would actually be able to sustain over time if you do make eating and exercise changes (Grilo 1996).

Maintaining Weight Loss

While weight loss is a challenging process, by far the more difficult stage is the maintenance of that loss. Perhaps even more dramatic than the role played by exercise during weight loss is its role during weight loss maintenance. In order to attain permanent weight control, changing your exercise patterns is at least as important as changing your eating habits. How much and what kind of exercise is necessary is still not entirely clear. And the reinforcing effect of persistence *per se* may be a major contributing factor. Nonetheless, one of the most accurate predictors of weight loss maintenance is the maintenance of exercise (Brownell 1994; Kirschenbaum 1994). "Increasing exercise may be the single most important thing an individual can do to lose weight and keep it off" (Kirschenbaum 1992, p. 83).

Exercise Recommendations for Weight Regulation

What kind of exercise will help you with weight loss? That's going to depend on you as an individual. Certainly, aerobic activity, because it efficiently increases your heart rate and metabolism, will be optimal on the "calories out" side of the equation. But getting moving is the first step, regardless of how vigorous it is.

Check It Out

If you are overweight, it will be important to review with your health-care provider your health status and any physical limitations before embarking on any strenuous activity. Although you may feel uncomfortable initiating such a discussion, most health-care providers will be very supportive of any interest that you have in increasing your level of physical activity.

Been There, Done That

If you are overweight, you have probably heard the exercise prescription more times than you can count. Like every diet that you've been through, this is very old news. That probably means that your values and beliefs about yourself and physical activity are fairly low. Understanding the value of exercise from a new and different angle may help you overcome your resistance to a recommendation that you've tried many times before—and feel like you've failed at. I hope that the information in this book about the many and varied benefits of exercise can help you take a different view of exercise in your life.

Feeling One Down

When you imagine yourself in comparison to all the "beautiful people" at the gym, you may anticipate feeling especially self-conscious about your looks and weight. Here are some ways to deal with this concern:

- Think about a comparable situation: when you see an adult with orthodontic braces, what do you think to yourself? Are you judgmental about their crooked teeth? If you're like me, you silently celebrate with them, pleased that they're taking care of their teeth.

- Be clear about *your* motives for exercise and keep those in mind. The best performers—athletes, musicians, and the like—focus on their own strengths rather than becoming distracted by others' performance. Your goals are not reflected in someone else's body.

- Think through more exactly what it is that you feel uncomfortable about. "Locker room anxiety" affects many of us. Sometimes it's a way to focus all our anxiety about starting something new and being with people we don't know. There may be ways around it. Would you feel more comfortable starting a class with a friend? What if you went to the gym with your exercise clothes already on?

- Feeling self-conscious is an utterly human trait. It is our way of attempting to protect ourselves from feeling rejected. But when these thoughts and feelings stop us from activities that we like and wish to do, or ones that will make us feel better, the price is too high. When you understand and accept your own concerns and at the same time develop creative solutions, you will feel stronger and more capable.

EXERCISE: WHAT'S SO SCARY?

What is your discomfort about exercise? How could you handle it?

I am uncomfortable about exercising because:

To handle that discomfort, I can:

_____   _____

_____   _____

_____   _____

_____   _____

Keeping Tabs

Weight distribution changes with exercise (Brownell 1994; Kirschenbaum 1994). Take your body measurements—remembering to write them down—before beginning a regular pattern of exercise. These figures will provide an alternate measure to that derived from your bathroom scale. They also have the advantage of having less symbolic meaning and therefore are less likely to get you caught up in negative expectations about yourself. For some people, as fat turns to muscle, measurements change more rapidly and more predictably than weight. And, as your body weight becomes redistributed, your clothes will start to fit differently and you will become and appear leaner.

Along with developing and maintaining an exercise pattern as well as changing your eating habits and patterns, another predictor of maintenance of weight loss is ongoing record keeping. The fact of the matter is that it seems not to matter exactly *what* you keep track of—it's the keeping track, the paying attention, that counts. The particular method that you use is less important than the actual recording. When you keep track, you are reinforcing your behavior and thus increasing the likelihood that you will continue to do it.

JOURNAL TASK: TRACKING YOUR EATING AND EXERCISE

You can use your journal to track a number of effects simultaneously. Here are some examples:

1. You can keep a classic food journal with columns for date, time, and food consumed—and the amount and type of exercise you've engaged in.

2. If you're interested in understanding more about your emotional relationship to food, you can add columns to note whether you were or weren't hungry before you ate, whether you were or weren't hungry once you finished, and your mood.

3. Over time, review and reflect on this journal, summarizing so that you can understand the patterns affecting you.

Learning to "Just Say No": Exercise and Substance-Abuse Cessation

Put together "sport or physical activity" with "alcohol or beer or cocaine or . . .", and what image comes to mind? Probably it's the latest media account of a basketball player strung out on coke and going for detox or the football player who just wrapped his SUV around a tree. And if you're watching sports on TV, where's the connection? Well, if you pay attention to the commercial breaks, it becomes more apparent: Commercials glamorize the relationship between alcohol and sports. Consider how many beautiful women and manly men you've seen in beer commercials during football games, and you'll begin to see what I mean.

Usually when we think of physical activity and substance abuse, we connect sports with an increase in substance abuse. Here we'll look at the ways in which exercise can help in the *recovery* from substance abuse. How does this happen? Let me share an example with you:

■ *Brian's Story*

Brian, an energetic thirty-six-year-old, has been sober for five years. The son of an alcoholic father, he began drinking and smoking marijuana in junior high school, was expelled from school, and did a stint in the army. He completed college and joined the family business, all while continuing to drink heavily and use a variety of drugs. He sobered up following a serious car accident, and agreed to hospitalization for detoxification. He became involved with AA at the time and started riding a bike.

Over the years, Brian has continued to be active in AA—he now is a regular sponsor for people just beginning the road to sobriety. He joined a bicycle club that holds weekly rides as well as occasional races. More recently, he joined a health club and has become an avid racquetball player. Along the way, he has also stopped smoking.

Given the great success of AA, no doubt Brian's attendance and involvement has contributed greatly to his sobriety. At the same time, there are six separate but interrelated reasons why his physical activity may be an important factor in his abstinence as well:

- **Physiological.** Although difficult to measure, positive biochemical changes are connected with exercise. At a physiological level, Brian may have been able to substitute the chemical effects of exercise for those of the various substances he had previously used.

- **The "synergy effect."** Good health habits cluster together, and one positive health behavior supports and increases the likelihood of another.

- **Distraction.** Both drinking and using substances take time. If you fill your time with activities such as exercise, you take up some of the "slack" that was previously occupied by substance use.

- **Sociability.** Brian is an outgoing man who enjoys being with people. Through the biking club and the health club he's joined, he has found new friends with whom to have fun. This is a different crowd than his former "drinking buddies." Brian has been able to establish a new, nondrinking identity, rather than returning to earlier peer pressures, expectations, and atmosphere.

- **Focus and outlet for emotions.** Brian is usually very tense and competitive. Working out hard, whether competing against himself or others, is a way he can channel this energy.

- **Mastery.** For many years, Brian thought of himself as unworthy and inadequate. He has been surprised and pleased with his skill development in biking and racquetball. He has enjoyed a sense of accomplishment. In addition, the sustained effort and commitment that he makes toward exercise serves to reinforce his sense of competence in continuing to refrain from drinking.

Alcohol and drug problems are major health and mental-health problems. About 10 percent of adults in the United States have significant problems with alcohol, and one-fourth of American adults regularly use tobacco (Miller and Brown 1997). Also, alcohol problems often occur among people with other mental health issues. It's been estimated that one-half of clients treated for medical or psychological problems have significant alcohol or other drug involvement.

Alcoholics Anonymous, as we saw with Brian, is an important route to sobriety. For some people, though, it's not only *not* sufficient, but there are actually aspects of AA that some people dislike. Recently, I spoke with my colleague Frieda, a sixty-one-year-old psychologist and self-described recovering alcoholic:

▪ *Frieda's Story*

Frieda is now in her twenty-first year of continuous sobriety. As far as she is concerned, drinking is no longer an option. It would be like driving a car without a seat belt, biking without a helmet, or wearing poor shoes when running. One just doesn't do these things, she feels.

In 1972, Frieda's doctor told her, dramatically, that she had to start exercising or she would die. At that point, she had been drinking heavily for years. Frieda took up running and enjoyed it so much that she began racing. Yet because of blackouts from drinking, she slept in and started missing races. She was furious with herself. Not getting to run in races was what finally convinced her to join AA. Ultimately, Frieda concluded that "AA is great for the beginner but all the #$%^ cigarette smoke and Lord's Prayer were 'turnoffs' for me. I disengaged after I had survived that critical first year. But I also don't think AA alone would have been sufficient.

"Running got me sober and has kept me sober. I run because of the joy of running, the poetry of the sunrise."

The desire to participate in road races rather than miss them through unconsciousness was what brought my colleague to sobriety. George Sheehan, a physician who was passionate about running, wrote a number of eloquent essays that speak to the mind-body connection. He also disclosed his own history of alcoholism:

Distance running ... was a positive factor and the decisive one. Negative injunctions never work. Lives are changed by do's, not don'ts. And if one is to stop drinking permanently, one must be actively involved in becoming what one is. Distance running did that for me. It reintroduced me to my body. And my body, I found out, had a mind of its own. It would no longer accept anything less than the best. ... Having reached the peak of its powers, it dragged my mind and my will along with it. (1978, p. 49)

Much of what we know about the relationship between exercise and sobriety is provided through stories, testimonials, and anecdotes. Only a few research studies have been conducted. These support the conclusion that exercise can be one important aspect of getting and staying on the wagon. When male college students who were heavy social drinkers participated in either an aerobic exercise or meditation program, they significantly reduced their alcohol consumption, equivalent to drinking fourteen fewer drinks per week (Murphy, Pagano, and Marlatt 1986). This program wasn't for everyone: 50 percent of the group dropped out during the experiment. Yet even when they did not look forward to running or meditation, the students noted in their journals that they felt less tense and much more relaxed, had an increased sense of well-being, and slept better after running or meditation. This behavioral change was apparently related to a number of elements: the opportunity for time out, time to themselves, a sense of accomplishment, and increased self-worth.

Exercise is frequently one aspect of inpatient recovery treatment. Various studies have found that with programs of physical exercise in place, not only is abstinence improved, but there is a decrease in anxiety, depression, and stress (Kremer, Malkin, and Benshoff 1995; Powers, Woody, and Sachs 1999; Sinyor, Brown, Rostant, and Seraganian 1982). The value of constructive use of leisure time, both as activity in itself and as an alternative to alcohol or drug use, has been emphasized repeatedly.

William Glasser, a psychiatrist, was one of the earliest to focus on the positive interaction of exercise and substance-use reduction (1976). He popularized the idea that "positive addiction" could be used as a substitute for "negative addiction." Broadly defined, he said that positive addiction helps strengthen people and facilitates increased life satisfaction. Negative addictions such as substance abuse, in contrast, weaken people and may "destroy" them. He suggested that what he called the "physical addictions," such as running, might be especially beneficial in discontinuing alcohol or smoking. He gave the following example: in response to a questionnaire Glasser had developed, a former "almost hopeless alcoholic" businessman who had stopped drinking now felt that running had completely "destroyed" any desire to drink. The man commented in relation to running: "I am always energetic and enthusiastic. I think quicker and clearer. I always feel like I always wanted to feel by having a few drinks" (p. 120).

In a survey of more than 700 readers of *Running Times*, one researcher noted a significant decrease in concern about addictions—alcohol, drugs, and/or cigarettes—over time for both men and women. With the exception of one woman, "the men and women who had begun to run in order to kick alcohol or nicotine dependency made it" (Johnsgard 1989, p. 47).

The Adventure Network near Philadelphia offers various combinations of adventure-based counseling and outdoor education, utilizing the challenge and enterprise inherent in group activities such as ropes courses, caving, rock climbing, and kayaking. One of its programs in particular, Adventures in Sobriety, is offered to people involved in Twelve Step programs, rehabilitation drug and alcohol centers, and high school and college groups. Therapeutic recreation professionals have created a national network, Therapeutic Recreators for Recovery, and provide both inpatient and outpatient therapeutic recreation programs, including walking, games, sports, weight training, and aerobics.

In addition to exercise as an aspect of recovery from substance abuse, exercise may be effective in preventing such problems. Danish, Nellen, and Owens (1996) pointed to an interactive cluster of health-compromising behaviors in adolescents, including drug and alcohol abuse, violent and delinquent behaviors, dangerous sexual practices, and school dropout. Yet potentially, primary prevention can disrupt this budding negative cluster. By acquiring life skills associated with success and learning health-enhancing behaviors, adolescents can learn "what to say yes to" (Danish, Nellen, and Owens 1996, p. 208). For them, activity can become a metaphor for enhancing competence.

Exercise Recommendations for Substance-Abuse Cessation

If you are recovering from a substance abuse problem, a regular and consistent program of physical exercise can be an important aspect of your recovery. Among other things, exercise will be able to help with:

- Distraction from your withdrawal symptoms or preoccupation

- Attention to your health and recovery

- Positive biochemical effects

- A sense of mastery and persistence

- The management of social isolation, and

- Stress and mood regulation.

- -

EXERCISE: MAKING IT PERSONAL (SUBSTANCE-ABUSE CESSATION)

Exercise helps me in my recovery because: _____

_____

_____

_____

- -

Many people starting a recovery program are not in good shape physically. Poor conditioning as a result of years of drinking or drug ingestion, as well as a lifestyle involving little exercise and poor nutrition, may be problematic. More serious damage to your heart, lungs, and/or liver is also a possibility. Therefore, it will be important to get full health clearance before starting any strenuous physical activity.

Walking may be an especially helpful form of exercise. Walking allows you to build up strength and enjoy the pleasures of being outdoors. It's also an activity that can easily be done with others, giving you opportunities for spending time with people in a way unrelated to addictive substances.

Exercise and Smoking Cessation

Now forty-four, Tina reflected on her exercise journey:

◼ *Tina's Story*

Regular exercise began when Tina was a college student. She was an over-weight smoker, "but still one of those adolescents with an immortality complex." One day in early spring a woman friend challenged her to run a mile. She took the challenge, ran the mile, collapsed at the end, and realized just how out of shape she was.

To her surprise, "I actually liked the feeling of running and took it up regularly. A short while later, I experienced a personal trauma, and exercise became an important way to deal with it. Running and swimming became my personal ways to feel control and power over my life, my self. So I ran with it."

Longtime running physician George Sheehan often wrote of the multiple benefits and interactions of exercise and other health habits. His perspective was that:

The athlete doesn't stop smoking and start training. He starts training and finds he has stopped smoking. The athlete doesn't go on a diet and start training. He starts training and finds he is eating the right things at the right time. (1978, p. 56)

Sometimes this shift occurs naturally. For other people, an obvious "wake up call" nudges them to make major health care changes:

◼ *Jonathan's Story*

Running to catch a bus, almost missing it, and severely out of breath, Jonathan wondered if he was having a heart attack. As his heartbeat slowed and he regained his composure, he flung away his cigarettes, vowing he would stop smoking. That evening he embarked on a program of running on a daily basis. Some twelve years and ten marathons later, he has continued not to smoke and finds it hard to remember his former self.

In a random survey of marathoners who had previously smoked, 81 percent of the men and 75 percent of the women stopped smoking when they began running. For men, there was a correlation between probability of smoking cessation and weekly mileage (Crandall 1986). And William Glasser, in his book *Positive Addictions* (1976), recognized the interrelatedness of constructive habits. He wrote of a man who had quit a two to three pack per day habit four months into running and suggested that running was as incompatible with smoking as it was with worrying.

A more matter-of-fact explanation about this connection is that people quit smoking because it interferes with their lung capacity and endurance once they've started to exercise. But which is the chicken and which the egg may be an individual experience.

Exercise Recommendations for Smoking Cessation

If you're in the process of quitting smoking, starting to exercise can be very helpful for a number of reasons:

- Many people don't quit smoking because they fear weight gain. (Nicotine is an appetite suppressant.) Since exercise burns calories and assists in the metabolic shift to a lower "set point" or weight balance, exercising can offset the typical increased poundage.

- Because exercise requires full lung capacity, the way in which you breathe when you exercise can serve as a good indicator of how well your lungs are recovering from the effects of smoking.

- Exercise can provide some of the mood-enhancing effects that you previously obtained from nicotine.

- If you are in the process of changing a health habit—whether it's losing weight, discontinuing alcohol or other substances, or quitting smoking—your persistence in exercise can help underscore your commitment to your overall improved health.

EXERCISE: MAKING IT PERSONAL (SMOKING CESSATION)

Exercise helps me in my recovery because: _____

_____

_____

_____

_____

As we've seen when discussing exercise, changing any health habit is a complicated process involving various stages of change (see chapter 3). Habits that are developed or maintained to avoid or diminish discomfort are among the most challenging to change. We've been discussing just those issues in this chapter—so if you're working on weight management or getting off substances, please recognize that this work *is* a big deal. Hopefully, with the addition of exercise, your path will feel more manageable.

CHAPTER 12

BEING FEMALE, BEING ACTIVE

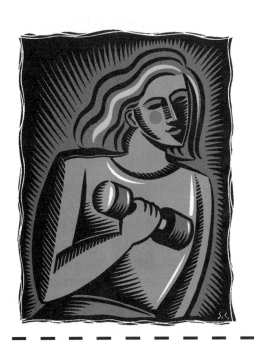

What does it *mean* to be a woman in relation to sport or exercise? The history of our knowledge about women and sport, like that of much scholarly research, has been that of generalizing from the experience of male sport participants to all sport participants (Bredemeier et al. 1991; Cogan and Petrie 1996; Duda 1991). This is a problem for research in general, but it's especially unfortunate and inappropriate when people study this particular topic. Traditionally, males, masculinity, and sports are equated; "women" and "sports" are often seen as unrelated categories.

The physical meaning of gender has been strikingly different, as well. Masculinity has been associated with energy, strength, and motion, while femininity has been associated with passivity, limitation, and protection. When men are concerned about body image, they usually focus on size and strength; female concerns typically relate to appearance (weight and slenderness) (Rindskopf and Gratch 1982). Boys consider that excess weight relates to muscle—and declare this a good thing; girls attribute excess weight to fat—and feel it's a bad thing. And if males want to lose weight, they typically increase exercise. Women, on the other hand, will start a new diet. When appearance is the definition of value as it often is for women, the capacity to age gracefully or with a sense of competence is undermined.

The early 1970s saw the beginning of the most recent wave of women's engagement in physical activity. The women's movement, Title IX (1972), and the development of the Women's Sport Foundation (1974) created an atmosphere for women's reclamation of their bodies and a surge in interest in understanding women's experience in sport and exercise. Yet even today, girls and women tend to be more sedentary and less involved in physical activity, as well as less engaged in organized, competitive sport than boys and men are (Duda 1991).

There is a paradox here: exercise is especially valuable for women but seemingly underappreciated by them. Female gender is one of the predictors of lack of exercise initiation (Dishman 1994). Lack of modeling, lack of social supports from friends or family, and a culturally prescribed attitude of selflessness are further barriers. Each of these issues is the direct opposite of those factors critical to the adoption of exercise (Sallis et al. 1992).

Let's review the benefits and barriers to exercise for women. We'll discuss the physical and psychological benefits—and look at some of the constraints as well.

Physical Benefits of Exercise for Women

In addition to the many physical benefits of exercise for the population as a whole, such as decreased risk for coronary heart disease, hypertension, and colon cancer (United States Department of Health and Human Services 1996), exercise also impacts more specifically female-related concerns such as PMS, menopause, osteoporosis, breast cancer, muscle mass loss, and weight management.

In a scathing critique of the use of psychotropic medications for premenstrual dysphoria, Prior, Gill, and Vigna (1995) instead encouraged the prescription of aerobic exercise. After a three-month program of mildly increasing exercise, they found that women experienced decreased fluid retention and breast tenderness. Following six months of minimal regular physical activity, their mood symptoms decreased. The authors commented,

> Why test an expensive drug when an inexpensive change in lifestyle, free of side effects and with positive effects on cardiovascular disease and the risk of osteoporosis, can be expected to provide benefit. . . . Science thinks it must rescue women from their bodies . . . more evidence of the negative view this culture holds of women and their physiology. (p. 1152)

Steege and Blumenthal (1993) compared the effects of randomly assigned aerobic exercise and (anaerobic) strength training on the premenstrual syndrome symptoms of twenty-three healthy premenopausal women (forty-five to fifty-five). Within three months of exercise participation, they found that both types of exercise served to reduce some PMS symptoms. Aerobic exercise, but not strength training, appeared to decrease depressive symptoms and more of the PMS symptoms. Preliminary findings in the Study of Women's Health Across the Nation (SWAN) suggest that, regardless of ethnicity, menopausal women who report getting less physical activity describe more estrogen-related and somatic symptoms (symptoms related to the body) (DeAngelis 1997). In contrast, exercise appears to be associated with decreased severity of hot flashes, although it is not clear whether this is a direct effect or mediated through the mechanism of diaphragmatic breathing (Barbach 1994).

Psychological Benefits of Exercise for Women

Along with the various physical benefits of exercise for women in particular, the psychological benefits may be even more significant. Women and girls can develop new body perceptions, ones that are less traditionally "feminine," yet still female.

> When exercise is strenuous, appearance is deemphasized. The sweatiness, labored breathing, tangled hair and facial grimaces that accompany hard physical exertion become part of the everyday experience. A new sense of body strength is gained as muscles replace fat and are capable of more and more work. Body competence is discovered as the first continuous mile or miles is achieved. Physical risk-taking occurs and pain becomes a sign of progress rather than a signal to stop. Even clothing becomes increasingly functional. Although improved muscle tone and, often, weight loss affect appearance in an external sense, the changes described are primarily internal. A woman can begin to appreciate her body for its power and function, variables over which she has an exceedingly reasonable degree of control. (Rindskopf and Gratch 1982, pp. 20f.)

Other, more specific, psychological effects may relate to issues of depression and interpersonal connectedness. Exercise has various meaning for us at different ages. Let's look at each of these.

Women, Depression, and Exercise

Regardless of race, education, occupation, nationality, willingness to seek help or report symptoms, twice as many women as men experience unipolar depression (McGrath, Keita, Strickland, and Russo 1990). At any given time, in the U.S. 2 to 3 percent of men and 4 to 9 percent of women suffer from depression (Kahn and Fawcett 1993). The lifetime risk for major depressive disorder has been estimated as ranging from 5 to 12 percent in men; for women, it is estimated at 10 to 25 percent (Martinsen and Morgan 1997). Women receive 70 percent of the prescriptions for antidepressant medication. Further, there is a high risk of improper diagnosis and misuse of prescription drug use among women (McGrath et al. 1990).

A biopsychosocial perspective on depression (taking into consideration biological, psychological, and social implications) suggests that social, economic, biological, and emotional factors all contribute to this international statistic. Likewise, a sociocultural perspective (considering societal and cultural factors) recognizes that women are much less likely than men to consider exercise under any circumstances, let alone when they are depressed and experiencing symptomatic low energy and a decreased sense of initiative. Further, a focus on depressed feelings and passivity rather than mastery and action among depressed women (McGrath et al. 1990) would predict less likelihood of exercise.

In a controlled experiment on the relationship between exercise and depression, McCann and Holmes (1984) randomly assigned forty-three depressed undergraduate women to an aerobic exercise, relaxation, or no-treatment condition. Women in the exercise condition developed improved aerobic capacity, and their level of depression decreased significantly more than among women in the other two conditions. Could aerobic fitness be useful in preventing the onset of depression following prolonged psychological stress? Over a nine-week period, information was gathered about a group of female college students. Those who were not fit and had experienced high life stress became depressed. Those with low stress, regardless of fitness, and those who were highly fit did not develop depression. This information leads researchers to conclude that aerobic fitness may serve a preventive function as well as having the potential to moderate the relationship between stress and depression (Holmes 1993).

Women and Sociability: Connecting and Disconnecting

Considering the importance that relationships have for most women, the social support and connection that a number of exercise programs provide can be an important aspect of exercise adherence for many women.

▪ *Meg's Story*

When Meg moved to the same neighborhood as her close friend Christa, both figured that they'd finally be able to spend time with each other on a regular basis. But Meg's kids pulled at her, and the demands of Christa's new business tugged at her. Meg exercised regularly; Christa knew that she should. Christa called Meg one Friday morning and said, "Let's go for a walk." Meg ran the mile to Christa's house, then they walked the two and a half mile loop around the neighborhood together. The hour they'd spent together in intimate conversation and movement felt like a gift. They decided to do it again the next Friday—and continued on, regardless of the weather, nearly every week for the next twelve years—until Meg moved away. Now, four years later, both will tell you that on Friday mornings, there's an empty hole.

Their conversation was that which occurs between two close women friends who know and respect each other's complex lives: work, child rearing, relationships, sense of self, and the ups and downs of their relationship with each other.

Meg incorporated the run plus walk into her regular routine of exercise. For Christa, the walk became a "call" to movement and connection. At times, she would find another friend with whom to walk, or she would do stretches or yoga by herself. The Friday walk was her steady, predictable time of movement and connection with her friend.

In part *because* of the ways in which relationships with others are vital for women, one of the particular values of exercise for some women is the opportunity for legitimate *dis*connection. Exercise can be the opportunity for social contact, or it can offer one a valuable time of privacy. Women overburdened with child-care responsibilities or "merely" the social commerce of life may experience legitimate solitude as a sought-after luxury.

■ Toni's Story

Having wrested a few precious moments from the demands of child care and work, Toni felt a special sense of triumph one day when the swimming pool at her gym was nearly empty. Paraphrasing Virginia Woolf, she appreciated having "a lane of my own."

In addition to the various benefits, there are different interactions at various age levels. Let's look at those next.

Girlhood and Adolescence

Along with the light blue and sweet pink of baby clothes, the ways in which boys and girls are socialized in relation to their bodies and activity are very different. We may have come a long way, but still parents will encourage boys to roam freely but be protective of little girls. Parents will even throw a ball differently, depending on whether it's to their one-year-old boy or their one-year-old girl. Not surprisingly, boys' and girls' attitudes about and involvement in sports is evident from an early age (Cogan and Petrie 1996; Eccles and Harold 1991). For example, by first grade, despite essentially comparable skills, girls feel significantly less competent in sport than do boys. Not surprisingly, they also are protective of their own egos: they feel markedly less invested in the sport domain than do boys and see sports as less important than other areas, such as academics (Eccles and Harold 1991).

The Title IX Act was designed specifically to create fiscal gender balance in sports, guaranteeing equal government funding for boys' and girls' sports. Although this sweeping federal legislation should, twenty-five years later, offset cultural biases and stereotypes, the impact and effectiveness of this act continues to be mixed (Duncan 1997). Certainly, more young girls are involved in organized sports. The phenomenal success of the 1999 U.S. Women's Soccer Team at the World Cup sparked an immense amount of interest and enthusiasm for that game and, more broadly, for women's legitimate involvement in competitive sport. Yet it's not clear whether the momentum created in younger years can override the societal constraints of adolescence. Can a young woman see herself as both female *and* an athlete? Perhaps. A high school basketball player, for example, said: "The court is where you can be all those things we're not supposed to be: aggressive, cocky, strong" (Blais 1995, p. 229). But when Victoria Bacon, a Boston-area sport psychologist, interviewed collegiate women athletes, they reported significant role conflict (Bacon 1997). The exciting news, though, was that these women reacted to this experience with a feeling of anger rather than withdrawal or shame. They recognized that there was a problem, but saw it as an issue of society rather than a conflict within themselves.

In the past few years, research has focused on the ways in which exercise may have an important impact on the lives of adolescent girls. A recent report by the President's Council on Physical Fitness and Sports (Physical Activity 1997) summarizes much of this research. While physical activity generally is associated with improved self-esteem and body image, the relationship is not uniformly straightforward for adolescent athletes, especially those involved in sports in which weight or appearance are relevant elements (Wiese-Bjornstal 1997). Among Caucasian females, athletes have lower school dropout rates and are more positively disposed toward the sciences than their nonathlete peers (Duncan 1997). Reviewing mental-health issues for adolescent females, Doreen Greenberg and Carole Oglesby (1997) have extended the research that exists for adults. They suggest that exercise therapy may offer a cost-effective and actively utilized treatment alternative or an adjunct to traditional psychotherapy or antidepressant drugs for young women experiencing depression or post-traumatic stress disorder.

The interaction of exercise and bone mass is important, complex, and perhaps age-related. While on the one hand, early exercise patterns can assist the development of bone mass, young women engaged in continual strenuous exercise are at higher risk for the "female athlete triad" of amenorrhea (lack of monthly menstruation), disordered eating, and osteoporosis (Freedson and Bunker 1997). The value of weight-bearing exercise or resistance training for the maintenance of bone mineral density and the prevention of osteoporosis in later years has been well established (Crandall 1986). The specific mechanisms are still being explored, as well as the intriguing question of whether exercise can serve as an osteogenic stimulus—that is, actually increase bone mass (Barbach 1994; De Souza, Arce, Nulsen, and Puhl 1994).

Ourselves as Mothers

No, I'm not talking about soccer moms. How does pregnancy affect our sense of our own bodies? How does incorporating the role of "mother" into our sense of self affect our view of ourselves? What are the messages that we give our children—male and female—about the value and pleasure of physical activity throughout life? When one of my clients took up exercise, her children's view of her changed dramatically:

◼ *Lindsay's Story*

At age thirty-eight, Lindsay began exercising for a number of reasons: weight loss, emotional control (both anger and sadness), and anxiety management. After six months of walking and/or riding her bicycle on a daily basis, she felt entirely committed to exercise as part of her definition of herself. She paid continuous and careful attention to the ways in which exercise served to help moderate her mood and stress. A combination of revised eating behaviors, social support, psychotherapeutic insight, and exercise resulted in a loss of 100 pounds in a year. Much to her surprise, she had come to view herself as a person who exercises. Evidently her children began to see her the same way, because when a teacher asked students to write a sentence-completion task, her daughter responded: "My mother . . . exercises."

Graham, a twenty-two-year-old who just graduated from college, reflected on his mother's influence, his late adoption of exercise, and the conclusions about sport and life that he has derived from his activity. Although this is the story of a male in a "female" chapter, his mother provided a role model that he then adapted in his own way:

◼ *Graham's Story*

Graham grew up in a single-parent home. His mother ran daily and enjoyed the mental and physical benefits of exercise. Although she had never spoken directly to Graham about it, he wondered if his mother was disappointed that he didn't get involved in sports in high school. He had played a couple of sports in elementary and junior-high school but always felt uncoordinated and self-conscious.

With the beginning of college, Graham was ready to try a number of new activities. He discovered that even though many colleges recruit students for crew, a number of students don't learn to row until college. With ten other novice rowers, young men as inexperienced as he was, Graham decided to try rowing.

"It was difficult at first to get in shape. Luckily, rowing doesn't take all that much coordination in the beginning. By the time you need to work on technique instead of power and drive, you've got enough skill to make coordination easier."

Graham began to see and feel the results of his practice. After he had trained diligently through his first semester and winter break, Graham's coach assigned him to practice with the varsity rowers. "What kept me going to practices was trying to overcome the initial difficulty of rowing, to prove to myself that I could do it. I worked harder and harder and by spring I had made the varsity boat. My love for the sport grew even more once I got a taste of competition.

"There were many times when I thought about quitting. It was difficult waking up at 5:15 A.M. to go out on the water, going to bed while my friends were going out drinking, and dealing with the fatigue and strain that come with a grueling sport.

"Every day there were opportunities to give up or take the easy way out. But the only way to get stronger was not to give in and to push harder. You get a feeling afterward that makes it all worthwhile, a sense that you've accomplished something.

"Staying with rowing has been one of the most rewarding experiences of my life. The physical shape I'm in because of rowing has let me do many other things that I now enjoy, including kayaking, hiking, and biking. I have learned a determination that I can carry through to every facet of my life."

Adult and Aging Women

Even more than adults in general, older adults and older women in particular tend not to participate in any kind of regular physical activity. "Throughout the life span, women are less active than their male counterparts, so that by late life, only a small minority are adequately exercising to benefit their health and well-being" (Cousins 1996, p. 131).

Without role models, with strong negative expectations about exercise, and with a belief that "I'm too old," older women—who may be at particular risk for depression or osteoporosis—are among the most in need, the most likely to show benefit, *and* the least likely to become involved. Elderly women might exaggerate the dangers of exercise, underestimate their physical abilities, believe that exercise need decreases with age, lack appropriate role models, and lack knowledge concerning the health benefits of exercise. And yet, older women stand to gain more than almost any other population group through exercise. Exercise is likely to retard osteoporosis; it helps women maintain their sense of balance, which is critical in reducing the chance of a dangerous fall; and recent research suggests that exercise may protect women in particular from Alzheimer's disease and other forms of dementia (Laurin et al., 2001).

Older women who *do* engage in exercise programs are more tuned into the physical and mental health benefits, social interaction, and stress reduction and mastery effects of exercise than their younger peers (who are likely to focus on weight management) (Gill and Overdorf 1994). My client Barbara illustrates this point:

■ Barbara's Story

I started meeting with Barbara when she was seventy-four years old. She came to me to discuss the growing discomfort her hiatal hernia was causing, as well as some serious feelings of unease that she was sicker than she knew. At Barbara's insistence, her doctor had conducted a variety of diagnostic tests, all of which had proved negative. Barbara felt there was *something* wrong and was concerned that perhaps he still had not uncovered some obscure underlying cause. Barbara understood that the more uneasy she became about her throat discomfort and problems in breathing, the more the discomfort increased, but she wasn't quite sure what to do about it.

Long widowed, Barbara enjoyed the combination of independence and connection available in sharing a two-family house with her son and his family. She
took pride in her health and independence and on not being perceived as "old."

I spent some time teaching Barbara the techniques of slow, deep breathing
(see chapter 5) and suggested that she say to herself the cue word "relax" each
time she exhaled. I also encouraged her to find out about taking yoga classes.
With its emphasis on diaphragmatic breathing and careful but not anxious
attention to body signals, I thought yoga might support a different way for
Barbara to understand her concerns. I also advised her to obtain more information about hiatal hernias, so that her health problems would not seem quite so
mysterious to her. In conversation with her physician, I recommended that he
listen less dismissively to her—and that he provide her with more information.
He was certain that there were no other problems, but agreed that if he were
less impatient with Barbara, she might feel that her concerns were being heard
and thus might feel less anxious.

Using a videotape, Barbara began learning yoga. She continued to be anxious about her breathing. I commented that these problems sounded like they
were a combination of reflux from the hernia plus anxiety. Challenging her to
live up to her capacity for independence rather than helplessness, I expressed
concern that she was in danger of becoming a hypochondriac. Hypochondriasis
has been estimated to occur in 10 to 15 percent of older adults (APA 1997b). We
did some more work on relaxation and anxiety management, and I again
encouraged her to get information and speak with her physician.

I saw Barbara for a final follow-up session a month later. She said that she
was feeling quite well. The reflux was markedly diminished, and she saw that
reduction as directly related to decreased anxiety, particularly through doing
daily yoga on her own. She was about to start taking weekly classes from a
yoga instructor.

An articulate colleague, Edith, commented to me about the multiple interactions of
body, body image, movement, and the pleasures of returning to a much-loved form of
physical activity:

▣ Edith's Story

Continuing to practice as a psychologist at age sixty-eight, Edith has also
stayed active and involved in various forms of exercise over the years, including swimming, aqua aerobics, yoga, t'ai chi, and walking.

As a young woman, she had been passionate about dance. But getting
older made her feel that she had to let it go: she assumed dancing was for a
certain sort of youthful, lithe body. Six months ago, however, she joined an
intergenerational dance group and now regularly rehearses and performs with
them.

Edith reflected on the many forms and functions of exercise: "Exercise
keeps me aware of my body in a very realistic way. I know what my body can
do and what it cannot do. I know that I can change my body in certain ways. I
can improve my flexibility and strength through yoga. I know that I can relax it
through t'ai chi and yoga.

"We get hung up on how our bodies look rather than what our bodies can do. What I am interested in learning about through this new dance experience is the aesthetic of the aging body, learning to give up some of the expectations that women have about their bodies."

Exercise Recommendations

Gender role socialization (that is, the ways we are brought up to understand what it means to be female or male) affects all of us. If you were raised before Title IX, you may be less likely to have a strong history of competitive sport to build on. Of course, there *can* be some advantages to a lack of experience in the sport domain. If or when you do start exercising, you may not have as many "ghosts" to fight as men often do. You may not have as many old memories to play off of, fewer impossible-to-attain expectations of yourself, and less identity attachment to a particular form or kind of exercise.

Back to the Future

Perhaps there are types of exercise you were involved with or wished to do as a child. These may be particularly compelling and empowering as you set out to increase your own sense of competence.

I started seeing Regina when she was sixty-four. Our initial conversation about exercise took her back to childhood and young adulthood:

> "What kind of activity did you enjoy when you were a child?" I asked her. Regina loved figure skating. She skated well into her twenties, though when she had children, she stopped. Would she be able to skate again someday? I asked. Regina seemed pleased at the prospect. As we discussed various forms of exercise—treadmill, swimming, biking—the image of herself skating again served as a guiding light. When she took her young grandchildren to skate, she knew that this year it wasn't possible—she needed joint replacement surgery—but perhaps next year. . . .

As I've described in this chapter, for many women, being physically active involves sorting out various concerns. Here are some Journal Tasks and Exercises to help you reflect and personalize the research and stories you've been reading.

Pumping Up

Researchers have repeatedly recognized that weight and strength training often enhances adolescent girls' and women participants' self-concept and body image (Gill 1995; Fisher and Thompson 1994; Wiese-Bjornstal 1997). (In addition, weight-bearing exercise is one of the most important preventatives of osteoporosis.) But some women feel uncomfortable with both the unfamiliar equipment and often male-dominated weight rooms in health clubs. You can ignore—or transform!—that atmosphere, or develop alternatives. The increasing number of women-only health facilities may be one ready solution. A fitness trainer, video, or book such as *A Woman's Book of Strength* (Andes 1995) can give you the fundamental tools you need to work out on your own at home.

JOURNAL TASK: PAST, PRESENT, AND FUTURE:

I REMEMBER WHEN . . .

In your journal, think back to your growing up years. You might write about these questions:

- What was my mother's attitude toward physical activity?

- How physically active was (or is) she?

- What was my family's attitude toward females being physically active as compared with males?

- How active was I as a child? As a teenager? As a young adult? What influenced me? What influenced decisions I made about physical activity?

- What activities did I love? What activities did I always want to do?

AND NOW. . . .

- How does my exercise history affect my current attitudes and behavior about exercise?

THINKING FORWARD

- How might these forms of exercise I identified be manifest in my life now?

- What kinds of social support will help me initiate and maintain activity?

- How can I reinforce my own sense of competence and self-efficacy for activity, and

- How can I justify for myself the value of taking time for my own needs?

JOURNAL TASK: DIALOGUE BETWEEN EXERCISE AND ME

Write a "dialogue" between you and Exercise (or Physical Activity) (or Sports). Think of Exercise as if it were alive, an actual being. See what it has to say to you—as well as what you want to say to it. As if you were writing a movie script, listen very carefully inside your head to "hear" this dialogue between parts of yourself.

JOURNAL TASK: LOOKING WITH DIFFERENT EYES

Review your Exercise History (chapter 4) and Cost-Benefit Analysis (chapter 3) particularly in light of gender issues. Think about what supports or challenges will arise if you take time for yourself to exercise.

As Karen Andes comments:

We're lucky that many of us are novices with weights. This makes us better students, blank slates, free from the burden of pride or past performance. We don't bring with us crusty old training methods and long-ingrained bad form or egos that need reassurance from hurling around heavy iron. (p. 7)

Grace and Balance

Balance and flexibility are other exercise results that have both physical and psychological benefits, particularly for women. As we get older, concern about and fears around falling can be of particular concern. Focusing specifically on balance and flexibility, through yoga, tai chi, or other Eastern arts, can be especially useful. The Eastern perspective also underscores and reinforces attention to our bodies as they currently are, rather than some idealized images.

A Final Note on the Subject

In the past number of years, as I return to run along streets and parks I've been before, it seems that more women—of many different sizes, shapes, and ages—are out there as well. It seems to me that we're out in greater numbers than ever before. I notice other women exercisers at Riverside Park in New York; I see them in the early morning light of the Mall in Washington, D.C.; two women stroll animatedly along the tree-shaded sidewalk of the suburbs of Boston. Is this a trend? It's hard to tell. Maybe the old ways are breaking up and women are coming into their own bodies. I hope so.

As we near the end of our work together, we will close the circle. Recognizing that at times exercise does not provide the complete solution to mental or emotional difficulties, we will look at the ways exercise can be combined with psychotherapy. And a final exercise is intended to help you reflect deeply on the meanings of exercise to your own well-being and sense of self.

PART 4

TAKING A "FEARLESS INVENTORY": REVIEW AND REFLECTION

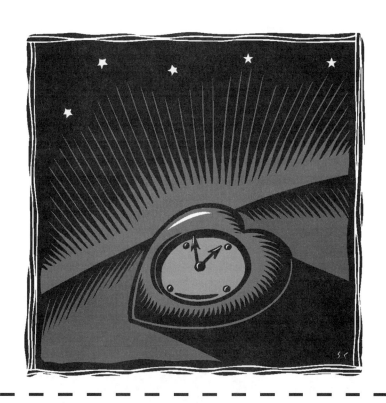

CHAPTER 13

WHEN EXERCISE ISN'T ENOUGH: EXERCISE AND THERAPY

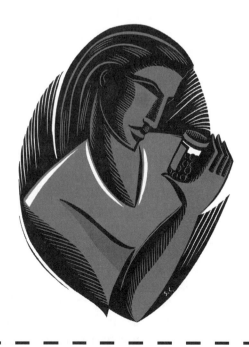

Exercise is an excellent means for feeling good and resolving any number of problems that confront us, but I fully recognize that it's not always enough. When you're feeling troubled, it can be extraordinarily useful to talk with someone else, someone who is neutral and not involved in your problems. But the choice doesn't have to be one or the other—either exercise or therapy. In this chapter, I bring together some thoughts about exercise *and* therapy. We'll look at the different ways exercise can be incorporated into therapy, the kinds of exercise that can be used during therapy, and why exercise and therapy, together, are helpful. But first, let's review what this chapter is *not* about.

Therapy Isn't Friendship: Setting Boundaries

Picture these situations:

- You know that your therapist is physically active and thinks exercise during therapy is helpful. Although you don't want to do it, you don't feel you can say "no" to your therapist, so you go along with her plan. (The therapy will be much more effective if you fully discuss your reluctance. The two of you can then decide to drop the topic altogether or revisit it at some other time.)

- You see your therapist at the health club to which you both belong. Both of you are squash players. "Wanna have a game?" either of you asks. (If you ask, your therapist should say, in a friendly way, "No. We have a different relationship that won't allow us to 'just play a game together.'" Your therapist should never ask in the first place.)

- You and your therapist have just come back from a therapy session in which you've both been physically active. It's a hot day and a beer would taste just great. "I brought along some beer. Wanna have some?" either of you asks. (Same scenario as above: your therapist should refuse, if you offer, and he or she should never be the one to make such a suggestion.)

- You and your therapist are both competitive recreational bike racers. One of you has a van; the other doesn't. A race is coming up next weekend. One of you says to the other: "Wanna carpool?" (You get the drift: If you ask, your therapist should refuse. And your therapist shouldn't offer—even if it *would* make your life easier.)

What do these scenarios say about the nature of therapy and the way that it's not the same as friendship? The first example is somewhat distinct from the other three: it emphasizes the power differential in therapy. In therapy, clients sometimes want to not disappoint their therapists. It is not uncommon (though it's neither appropriate nor useful) for clients to strive to please their therapists in ways that override their own thoughts, feelings, and needs. If this same situation happened with a friend, it might be fairly easy for you to decline the invitation—and talking about it might or might not be relevant to your friendship. One of the central *purposes* of therapy, often, is to help you sort out what your feelings are and potentially help you interact with people in a different way. Thus, declining (even if it's with some anxiety, self-doubt, and concern about how you'll be viewed) can actually be a therapeutic action *if* you and the therapist take the opportunity to deal with the interaction between the two of you.

The second example sets up a situation that is by definition competitive. Sometimes friendship contains an element of competitiveness. But therapy is designed to be about *you*. It makes no sense (and would be confusing, if not harmful) to deliberately add a layer of competitiveness to psychotherapy.

The third example is the "slippery slope." This one, the slide from the formal therapy relationship toward friendship (whether or not it contains an element of sexual attraction), is the primary reason why many therapists not only don't exercise with clients, but recognize the dangers that might be inherent in this activity. Again, it is the therapist's responsibility to monitor the boundaries of the relationship.

As for carpooling—well, why not? It's convenient. It's a friendly thing to do. But: what do you talk about in the van? Your problems? That would be free therapy. Your therapist's problems? How would that change what you say to your therapist in your subsequent sessions? Who pays for the gas? What does that mean? How do you introduce each other at the site? And so on. What might seem like a simple gesture can quickly become complicated.

Why Therapy?

Wait a second, you may be saying. This is a book about emotions and exercise, movement, and feeling good about yourself. How did psychotherapy get in here? Well, psychotherapy is one really important solution to feeling bad about yourself. Before talking about possible connections between exercise and therapy, let's talk about therapy itself.

Why would a person seek psychotherapy? Generally, you'd be interested in therapy if:

1. You're feeling troubled;

2. Your problems are frequent enough or intense enough or have persisted for long enough (yes, this is our FIT acronym once again) that some kind of intervention seems important;

3. Other resources, such as friends or family, reflection, journaling, or reading haven't sufficiently resolved the problems.

Problems come in all shapes and sizes. We've mentioned some of them, such as depression, anxiety, eating disorders, and so on. Problems also come in a variety of levels of seriousness. One measure of seriousness is how long problems have lasted. Another measure has to do with how uncomfortable the person feels about the problems or symptoms. And another relates to how much the problems interfere with a person's daily life and functioning.

Psychotherapy these days also comes in many shapes and sizes. Going back to Freud, there is the classic image of a person lying on a black couch spending years talking about their miserable childhood while a psychoanalyst nods sagely in the background. This kind of treatment, while still out there, is much less typical than the numerous variations now available. More commonly, the therapist and client sit facing each other, the client focuses more on their present concerns, and the therapist takes a somewhat active role in assisting the person in understanding what the issues are and what some solutions might be. Different therapies vary in terms of how much emphasis is placed on a person understanding their problems and how much energy is focused on ways of handling these problems. But in all forms of therapy, the quality of the relationship between the therapist and client, the way in which a client feels accepted and understood, forms the significant core (Whiston and Sexton 1993).

EXERCISE: WHAT DO YOU THINK OF THERAPY?

Even though more people are receiving therapy these days and more people are talking about their therapy experiences, many of us still feel uncomfortable when thinking about therapy as applied to ourselves. Write out some of your fears, concerns, or discomforts—and some reasonable answers you might give to those concerns.

Negative Thoughts about Therapy	*Rational Responses about Therapy*
EXAMPLE:	
Everyone will think I'm crazy if I go to a therapist.	My friend Will saw a therapist and he's not crazy. Besides, he's less worried and sleeps better now.
Therapy will be too expensive.	If it saves my relationship, it's worth the cost.

Working It Out: The Link Between Exercise and Psychotherapy

If exercise is going to be incorporated into psychotherapy in some way, it will depend on the interaction of three different aspects: you and your level of fitness or interest; the importance of exercise to the therapy session itself; and your therapist's role. Each of these characteristics can vary, from no involvement to extensive involvement. And it's not as if the situation were static, with therapy, or you, or your therapist feeling and acting exactly the same each time. For instance: over time, you may become more or less physically active. Or issues around exercise may become more or less relevant to the therapy. Or your therapist's role in this regard may shift as exercise issues become more or less important to you.

Let's start with you: You might be physically inactive, not currently exercising. In that case, you will be like most people starting psychotherapy—and like most people in North America. If you're already active and committed to exercise, there may be more options available for using exercise in psychotherapy.

And how might exercise be or become part of therapy? As we've seen throughout this book, exercise can be a "therapeutic," that is, good for you. Sometimes it's the best "prescription" for your mental health. More often, if you've got serious problems, exercise can be a powerful adjunct to psychotherapy. Exercise is not seen as the primary therapy—talking serves that function—but it is recognized and supported as helpful. Occasionally, exercise can be the medium in which the psychotherapy is practiced.

And what is your therapist's role in this process? Again, it may vary. If your therapist is knowledgeable about exercise and considers it appropriate within the bounds of therapy, he or she may consult with you about your own exercise: they might support or encourage exercise or offer you some technical or training advice. If they exercise, they might serve as something of a role model for you. If it makes sense in light of you and your needs, as well as your therapist's willingness and interest, your therapist might exercise with you during therapy.

Three ways that exercise and psychotherapy can be linked involve support, movement during an impasse, and the occasional use of exercise as the medium for psychotherapy. Since many of the case examples in this book involve the support and encouragement of exercise while a client is in psychotherapy, there is no need to repeat that information. We'll describe the other two methods briefly here.

Walking It Out vs. Waiting It Out: Using Exercise to Assist the Therapy

Therapy is an endlessly fascinating process. When it's going well, there's an interchange, an energy and flow of thoughts and ideas between the client and the therapist. But at times there may be an impasse: a client experiences so much anxiety or tension that he cannot do the work that he's there to do. Now, different therapists handle such a situation in a variety of ways—I do, too, depending on the client and the issue. Sometimes it's useful for the therapist to just wait out the situation. At other times, a therapist might ask about the meaning of the anxiety or make use of it as an occasion for a client to practice anxiety-management techniques. But there are times when none of these is likely to move the therapy forward: therapist and client sit, facing each other, the client becoming more anxious, withdrawn, immobilized, and silent. At some of those moments, I have suggested that we move outside the office to continue our session. Although other therapists no doubt use this method, not many have written about it. Dr. Wesley Sime of the University of Nebraska (one of the few who *has* written on the subject) says that in addition to recommending "walk-talk" therapy as a way to support exercise initiation, he also at times suggests walking during therapy when a client seems mired in silence. Similarly, Jon Kabat-Zinn (1990) describes a client at the University of Massachusetts Medical Center's stress reduction program whose already high level of somatic anxiety increased radically when she attempted to engage in the stillness of mindfulness training. It was only through walking meditation that she could begin learning methods for stress reduction.

With my client Shana, for example, going for a walk was an attempt to help a session become more productive:

▣ *Shana's Story*

Referred by her couples therapist for individual therapy, twenty-seven-year-old Shana, herself a therapist, was brittle and self-conscious throughout our sessions. She seemed to be continuously second guessing herself. "I feel dysfunctional and damaged," she commented. After four months of treatment, she was, if anything, even tighter and quieter than earlier. She was emotionally shut down, left sessions early, canceled appointments at the last minute, and when she was present, seemed unable to think of what to talk about. She stopped herself from talking, sure that I would see how "messed up" she was.

Rather than continuing to hope that we could work through or ride out the tension, I suggested during one session that we try walking as we spoke. Although there was initially much silence, as we walked she finally began to talk about a prior painful therapy experience.

Shana was already exercising regularly and finding it of value in decreasing her irritability. This in-session walk was not designed as a means to encourage exercise itself. It was a way of managing anxiety so that Shana would be able to do the work of therapy. We used this method one more time, again when she was extremely tense, and again she was more verbal, though still unsure about therapy.

Exercising During Therapy

There are a number of potential benefits of exercise occurring during psychotherapy. These include:

- The development or maintenance of the exercise habit,

- Access to feelings,

- Changes in thinking patterns,

- The use of symbolism and metaphor,

- Nonverbal communication.

Let's look at these in more detail.

If you're just beginning to exercise, exercising during therapy can support and reinforce the benefits of this activity. Moving during therapy, rather than only talking about being physically active, can be a motivator for more exercise at other times and places.

Exercise loosens up your mind as well as your muscles. You become more aware of various feelings, both those that are near the surface and those that may lie deeper. You feel less inhibited and less self-conscious about talking about these feelings and thoughts. You can talk about what you genuinely feel (in contrast to what you think you should feel). You are more *conscious* of yourself, but less *self-conscious*.

The qualities of thinking that are so satisfying about exercise for some people (see chapter 8) are exactly those that can be beneficial during therapy. Your thinking may feel clearer, or you may understand old problems in a new way. You are doing the "right brain problem solving" we discussed, integrating the two sides of your brain. You are fully utilizing your mind and body in the presence of someone who can guide you in that process, reinforce your insights, and help you explore more deeply. You feel more "centered." In a conversation, Dr. Sime commented on this process (personal communication, February 11 1998):

> A dramatic difference between exercise (walk-talk) therapy and traditional psychotherapy is that while walking side by side, there is very little face-to-face conversation. This indirect interaction may free up the client to be more spontaneous and thoughtful without regard to self-conscious concerns of appearance, behavior, and vocabulary. A client who might ordinarily feel uncomfortable in traditional psychotherapy tends to feel much more at ease or spontaneous in a discussion while walking simply because it has the appearance of being casual and unintimidating. Much like the exertional manifestations of deeper breathing and the more forceful expulsions of air in respiration, talking while walking elicits spontaneity.

Some Things for You to Consider

Exercise during therapy differs dramatically from traditional psychotherapy. The shared activity results in a more equal balance between therapist and client. Many of the issues involved in exercising during therapy are ones that your therapist should be clear about (such as interpersonal issues, training, and ethics). Interested therapists are referred elsewhere for further discussion on these topics (for example, Hays 1994, 1999; Sime 1996). The therapist always retains responsibility for creating and maintaining boundaries so that a harmful dual role relationship does not develop. For clients, there are both logistical and personal considerations.

Logistically, there are basic issues of organization and physiology: are changes of clothing required, and how are those handled? Are both of you sufficiently fit to carry on conversation while moving? Can you accommodate each other's pace—and converse at the same time? The greater the level of activity, the more relevant these questions become.

Are you able to use exercise as the medium in which psychotherapy occurs, rather than the focus of the therapy? This may be a function both of your fitness and the role of activity in your life.

To what degree does physical activity allow you to avoid particular emotions rather than confront them and work them through? Some therapists who are skeptical about exercise in therapy have asked this important question. In therapy, there is always a tension between containment and expression. Is therapy about controlling your thoughts and feelings or about developing greater openness? The answer to this question of course varies among different clients—even the same client at different times, or regarding different issues—and therapists with varied training and perspectives. My experience is that if anything, the medium of physical activity can allow the expression and resolution of feelings that otherwise are blocked from clients' awareness.

Walking During Therapy

Therapists who suggest exercise to their clients often recommend walking. When I've spoken informally with other therapists, it appears that if exercise is employed during therapy, it is most likely to be walking. Walking is safe for most people. As I described with Shana, it can be used as a method to decrease anxiety. A client and a therapist can maintain a dialogue while walking together. The logistics are fairly effortless and straightforward. And it may serve as the base for developing other exercise habits (Sime 1996). Also, because it's so ordinary and natural, walking seems less "different," less novel, and less complicated than running. And it may have some of the same mental benefits for therapeutic change. For example, after some months of in-office therapy, my client Phyllis and I conducted most of the subsequent therapy outside, walking:

▣ *Phyllis' Story*

Phyllis entered therapy with acute symptoms of major depression, panic disorder, vivid post-traumatic stress disorder (PTSD), and morbid obesity. For many years, overeating was the primary way she attempted to manage the other three symptom clusters. Her history involved severe, frequent, and long-standing physical and verbal abuse from her mother as well as violent sexual abuse by her brother.

Initially, I suggested exercise to Phyllis because of its biochemical capacity to decrease anxiety and depression. Exercise, I explained to her, was a powerful method for controlling panic and decreasing depression. Regular exercise would also be the most effective and healthy way that she could begin losing weight—one of her primary goals. As it turned out, the distraction of exercise also gave her better access to imagery as she resolved some of her traumatic early history.

Over a ten-month period, the use of a stationary bicycle and decreased binging resulted in a twenty-pound weight loss. This weight loss was sufficient to ease a chronic foot problem. Phyllis began going for occasional walks, and in the midst of a very difficult time, she suggested a few times that we walk for part of the therapy hour, which we did.

With the resolution of her history of severe physical and sexual abuse, Phyllis began feeling comfortable enough in her own body to undertake more intense weight-reduction efforts. In addition to dietary management and regular attendance at a community weight-management support group, she began walking on a systematic, daily basis. We started to walk routinely while conducting therapy, again at her suggestion. Initially, we walked for about twenty minutes of the session. Within two months we were walking the entire session, about two and a half miles each time. Phyllis increased exercise at home to about five miles a day, five to six days a week. Just as with stationary bicycling, walking now had a number of purposes: to sustain the weight loss, to regulate her mood, and to create time and means to think through issues.

Phyllis commented: "Pondering difficulties while I'm fully engaged in physical activity allows me to visualize new approaches. I feel 100 percent of me is free to engage my mind in solutions and possibilities. My mind feels less cluttered, and my thinking is unencumbered by negativity."

For the most part, the content of the therapy session was the same as it would have been in the office. Yet there were differences, too—metaphoric opportunities that could be experienced, understood, and spoken. Phyllis used the symbolism of her newfound strengths. As we began one session, she remarked: "Let's do hills today. I have stressful things to talk about." The effort of walking up a hill paralleled her internal challenges.

Running During Therapy

About twenty years ago, great enthusiasm and fanfare greeted the idea of running during therapy. Thaddeus Kostrubala, a psychiatrist in California, became a well-known advocate of this method of therapy (1977). Although there have been occasional references to it (for instance, California psychologist Keith Johnsgard wrote about running combined with therapy a decade later) little has been heard (or written) on this subject since then. Probably a number of reasons account for that: the excitement of the running fad has passed; we live in a litigious society, and therapists are rightfully cautious about trying techniques about which there isn't much information; and even though some therapists are doing this kind of therapy, they aren't writing about it. There is also the practical matter that if therapy is going to occur while running, both of you will need to be sufficiently fit to be able to run and talk at the same time.

Because I think that, with careful selection and a good match between therapist and client, this kind of therapy *can* be extremely useful, I'll share with you an example of the use of running during therapy.

▪ Polly's Story

Polly was a thirty-two-year-old doctoral student who taught at a small college. During adolescence, she informed the police of her father's twelve-year history of sexual assault on her, and he was arrested, tried, found guilty, and imprisoned. As is true of many incest survivors, Polly entered psychotherapy with a variety of effects from her history. Among other things, she experienced problems with intimacy, wasn't sure what the appropriate limits were in relationships, and was either very passive or too demanding. She was often emotionally overwhelmed and had difficulty integrating her thoughts, feelings, and actions. She experienced violent, terrifying nightmares, chronic disorganization of time and money, and significant lapses in recollection of her history.

Polly entered one session in such agitation that she could not sit still. She began pacing the room. It was a beautiful New England fall day, and I knew that Polly regularly engaged in various forms of strenuous exercise with a number of friends, so I suggested that we continue therapy while walking. She was immensely relieved at the suggestion, and as soon as we were outside, was again able to carry on with the session. We walked for about a mile. Polly commented favorably on the walk. I was intrigued by the seeming helpfulness of movement to her therapeutic process and asked whether she might be interested in trying a session while running. She was immediately enthusiastic.

We ran during most of the subsequent sessions, maintaining a pace that allowed us to talk. With a standard circuit of about three miles, there was enough time when we returned to the office for us to draw conclusions, summarize, and resolve any remaining issues.

Polly, who at times was reduced to inarticulate tears in the office, was able while running to experience, express, and understand her emotions. In a number of sessions, the increased capacity to observe as well as experience herself was strikingly evident. While this improvement may have been in part a function of length of treatment, the treatment medium also played a significant role.

Reflecting on the mind-body connection, Polly commented at one point: "Running during therapy feels like a very active form of learning. I process information through my body and from there to my mind, and then it gets integrated. The physical sensations are like a feedback loop that serves to validate and confirm my feelings. Sometimes part of the run is very difficult—the idea or issue we discuss may be difficult for me to grasp or upset me emotionally. When that happens my breathing and pulse increase, my stride shortens—all the symptoms of being physically stressed. During my athletic training, I've learned to 'listen' to the physical signs and respond accordingly—I try to slow the rate of my breathing, lengthen my stride, and run from a centered point in my body. My physical 'observer' has been active for a long time, and now I'm learning to listen to my emotions. I'm really at a point where awareness is important and being aware of my body has helped me be aware of my feelings." (Hays 1994, p. 732)

In this chapter, we've added more food for thought. That "food" might be the idea of therapy for you. Or it might be the idea of exercise in relation to therapy. When it comes down to the individual human being, psychotherapy is an art as well as a science, a practice in which you as active participant are as knowledgeable about you as your therapist is about problems and their solutions. Take some time to reflect on what you know about yourself and your own needs.

JOURNAL TASK: MY NEEDS
AND THEIR SOLUTION

This is an exercise that can be repeated numerous times. It is both a snapshot of a particular moment and a guide toward your future. Use the sentence stems, or write freely on the topics.

At present, my emotional needs are _____

At present, I am concerned about _____

I have addressed these issues by _____

I have received support from _____

Therapy might be useful for me if _____

I would be interested in therapy and exercise if _____

CHAPTER 14

A FINAL EXERCISE

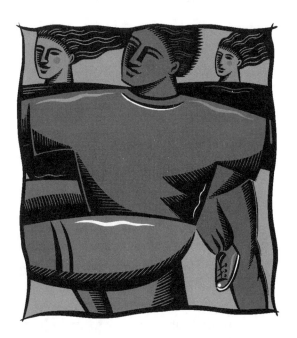

Now that we're coming to the end of our journey together, a final exercise can help you mark your current place and move toward a new sense of where you're going. As with many other exercises, this is one that you may wish to repeat at various relevant intervals.

EXERCISE: ON REFLECTION

Write a letter in which you consider what you've learned as you have been reading this book and the ways in which you now understand more about yourself and exercise. You can write this as:

1. A formal letter to yourself, complete with salutation and signature.

2. A formal letter to yourself-in-three-months, writing to your future self about your interest and involvement in exercise and your anticipations for the future. Put the letter in a self-addressed, stamped envelope, seal it, and give it to a friend whom you can trust to actually put the letter in the mailbox in three months.

3. An "unsent letter" addressed to me—that is, a letter that you decide ahead of time to *not* send. This allows you to write freely without censoring yourself in any way. Because it's addressed to someone else, the letter will have the additional energy we put into dialogue.

4. An actual letter to me (addressed to Kate Hays, c/o New Harbinger Publications, 5674 Shattuck Avenue, Oakland, CA, 94609).

In your letter, consider writing about some of the following:

1. Reading this book, I learned that _____.

2. Reading this book, I re-learned/became clearer that _____.

3. I found _____ especially relevant, but _____ had no particular meaning for me. I wish that there were more about _____. In order to get that information, I will _____.

4. This is my exercise story now.

Reading and reflecting, thinking and moving, planning and taking action—all of these involve different aspects of our being. As we have journeyed together through this book, you have had the opportunity to think about the meaning of exercise and the notion of changing your behavior. We've discussed exercise as a way to be therapeutic to yourself when you have specific problems or concerns. We've reviewed the challenges of becoming and staying motivated. We've even explored the hybrid of exercise and psychotherapy.

I've led you on this journey to assist you in getting on with your life in a healthy and meaningful way. If you've been tracking your mood when you exercise, you are understanding from within your very own being the pleasure and energy of physical activity. Appreciating and enjoying the natural benefits of exercise will go a long way toward helping you meet your goals and live a happier, healthier life.

Perhaps you've discovered the delicious sensation of stretched-out muscles. Maybe your walking and your thoughts are taking flight. You may know your direction, but still need metaphoric pausing points along the way, to catch your breath and attend to the scenery.

Whatever your journey, as you continue along your way I wish you activity and energy, thoughtfulness and a center of calm. This exploration is never-ending, yet always interesting and often exciting. Bon continued voyage!

REFERENCES

American Psychiatric Association. 1993. *Practice Guideline for Major Depressive Disorder in Adults.* Washington, D. C.: Author.

American Psychological Association. 1997. *Working with Older Adults* [Brochure]. Washington, DC: Author.

Andes, K. 1995. *A Woman's Book of Strength: An Empowering Guide to Total Mind/Body Fitness.* New York: Berkley.

Babyak, M. A., J. A. Blumenthal, S. Herman, P. Khatri, P. M. Doraiswamy, K. A. Moore, W. E. Craighead, T. T. Baldewicz, and K. R. Krishnan. 2000. Exercise treatment for major depression: Maintenance of therapeutic benefit at 10 months. *Psychosomatic Medicine* 62:633-638.

Bacon, V. L. 1997. Re-solving voice and the female college athlete. *Journal of Applied Sport Psychology* 9[Suppl]:S18.

Barbach, L. 1994. *The Pause: Positive Approaches to Menopause.* New York: Signet.

Bahrke, M. S., and W. P. Morgan. 1978. Anxiety reduction following exercise and meditation. *Cognitive Therapy and Research* 2:323-333.

Barlow, D. H. 1997. Cognitive-behavioral therapy for panic disorder: Current status. *Journal of Clinical Psychiatry* 58[Suppl 2]:32-37.

Benson, H. 1984. *Beyond the Relaxation Response.* New York: Berkley.

Berger, B. G. 1994. Coping with stress: The effectiveness of exercise and other techniques. *Quest* 46:100-119.

Berger, B. G., E. Friedman, and M. Eaton. 1988. Comparison of jogging, the relaxation response, and group interaction for stress reduction. *Journal of Sport & Exercise Psychology* 10: 431-447.

Berger, B. G., and R. Motl 2001. Physical activity and quality of life. In *Handbook of Sport Psychology* (2nd edition) edited by R. N. Singer, H. A. Hausenblas, and C. M. Janelle. New York: Wiley.

Beumont, P. J. V., C. C. Beumont, S. W. Touyz, and H. Williams. 1997. Nutritional counseling and supervised exercise. In *Handbook of Treatment for Eating Disorders*, edited by D. M. Garner and P. E. Garfinkel. New York: Guilford.

Blais, M. 1995. *In These Girls, Hope Is a Muscle.* New York: Warner Books.

Blumenthal, J. A., M. A. Babyak, K. A. Moore, W. E. Craighead, S. Herman, P. Khatri, R. Waugh, M. A. Napolitano, L. M. Forman, M. Appelbaum, P. M. Doraiswamy, and K. R. Krishnan. 1999. Effects of exercise training on older patients with major depression. *Archives of Internal Medicine* 159:2349-2356.

Booth, Frank W. 2001. *35 Conditions That Are Caused or Worsened by Inactivity* [online]. Available: www.ridinactivity.org/35_conditions.htm.

Bordo, S. 1993. *Unbearable Weight: Feminism, Western Culture, and the Body.* Berkeley: University of California Press

Bredemeier, B. J. L., G. S. Desertrain, L. A. Fisher, D. Getty, N. E. Slocum, D. E. Stephens, and J. E. Warren. 1991. Epistemological perspectives among women who participate in physical activity. *Journal of Applied Sport Psychology* 3:87-107.

Bruch, H. 1978. *The Golden Cage: The Enigma of Anorexia Nervosa.* New York: Vintage.

Cameron, J. 1992. *The Artist's Way: A Spiritual Path to Higher Creativity.* Los Angeles: J. P. Tarcher.

Casper, R. C., and L. N. Jabine. 1996. An eight-year follow-up: Outcome from adolescent compared to adult onset anorexia nervosa. *Journal of Youth and Adolescence* 25: 499-517.

Clayton, P. J. 1990. The comorbidity factor: Establishing the primary diagnosis in patients with mixed symptoms of anxiety and depression. *Journal of Clinical Psychiatry* 51:11[Suppl]:35-39.

Cogan, K. D., and T. A. Petrie. 1996. Diversity in sport. In *Exploring Sport and Exercise Psychology*, edited by J. L. Van Raalte and B. W. Brewer. Washington, DC: American Psychological Association.

Cousins, S. O. 1996. Exercise cognition among elderly women. *Journal of Applied Sport Psychology* 8:131-145.

Crandall, R. C. 1986. *Running: The Consequences.* Jefferson, NC: McFarland and Co.

Csikszentmihalyi, M. 1990. *Flow: The Psychology of Optimal Experience.* New York: Harper and Row.

Danish, S. J., V. C. Nellen, and S. S. Owens. 1996. Teaching life skills through sport: Community-based programs for adolescents. In *Exploring Sport and Exercise Psychology*, edited by J. L. Van Raalte and B. W. Brewer. Washington, DC: American Psychological Association.

Davis, C., S. H. Kennedy, E. Ralevski, M. Dionne, H. Brewer, C. Neitzert, and D. Ratusny. 1995. Obsessive compulsiveness and physical activity in anorexia nervosa and high-level exercising. *Journal of Psychosomatic Research* 39:967-976.

Davis, M., E. R. Eshelman, and M. McKay. 2000. *The Relaxation and Stress Reduction Workbook.* Oakland, CA: New Harbinger.

DeAngelis, T. 1997. Menopause symptoms vary among ethnic groups. *APA Monitor*, November, 16.

De Souza, M. J., J. C. Arce, J. C. Nulsen, and J. L. Puhl. 1994. Exercise and bone health across the life span. In *Women and Sport: Interdisciplinary Perspectives*, edited by D. M. Costa and S. R. Guthrie. Champaign, IL: Human Kinetics.

Diener, E. 2000. Subjective well-being: The science of happiness and a proposal for a national index. *American Psychologist* 55:34-43.

Dimeo, F., M. Bauer, Varahram, G. Proest, and U. Halter. 2001. Benefits from aerobic exercise in patients with major depression: A pilot study. *British Journal of Sports Medicine* 35:114-117.

Dishman, R. K. 1988. Overview. In *Exercise Adherence*, edited by R. K. Dishman. Champaign, IL: Human Kinetics.

———. 1994. Introduction: Consensus, problems, and prospects. In *Advances in Exercise Adherence,* edited by R. K. Dishman. Champaign, IL: Human Kinetics.

Duda, J. 1991. Editorial comment. *Journal of Applied Sport Psychology* 3:1-6.

Duncan, M. C. 1997. Sociological dimensions. In *Physical Activity and Sport in the Lives of Girls: Physical and Mental Health Dimensions from an Interdisciplinary Approach*. Rockville, MD: SAMHSA.

Eccles, J. S., and R. D. Harold. 1991. Gender differences in sport involvement: Applying the Eccles' expectancy-value model. *Journal of Applied Sport Psychology* 3:7-35.

Epling, W. F., and W. D. Pierce. 1991. *Solving the Anorexia Puzzle: A Scientific Approach*. Toronto: Hogrefe and Huber.

Etnier, J. L., W. Salazar, D. M. Landers, S. J. Petruzzello, M. W. Han, and P. Nowell. 1997. The influence of physical activity, fitness, and exercise upon cognitive functioning: A meta-analysis. *Journal of Sport and Exercise Psychology* 19:249-277.

Fairburn, C. G. 1995. *Overcoming Binge Eating*. New York: Guilford.

Fisher, E., and J. K. Thompson. 1994. A comparative evaluation of cognitive-behavioral therapy (CBT) versus exercise therapy (ET) for the treatment of body image disturbance: Preliminary findings. *Behavior Therapy* 18:171-185.

Foreyt, J. P., and G. K. Goodrick. 1992. *Living Without Dieting*. New York: Warner.

Freedson, P., and L. K. Bunker. 1997. Physiological dimensions. In *Physical Activity and Sport in the Lives of Girls: Physical and Mental Health Dimensions from an Interdisciplinary Approach*. Rockville, MD: SAMHSA.

Gallwey, W. T. 1997. *The Inner Game of Tennis*. Revised ed. New York: Random House.

Gill, D. L. 1995. Gender issues: A social-educational perspective. In *Sport Psychology Interventions*, edited by S. M. Murphy. Champaign, IL: Human Kinetics.

Gill, K., and V. Overdorf. 1994. Incentives for exercise in younger and older women. *Journal of Sport Behavior* 17:87-97.

Glaros, N. M. and C. M. Janelle. 2001. Varying the mode of cardiovascular exercise to increase adherence. *Journal of Sport Behavior* 24:42-62.

Glasser, W. 1976. *Positive Addiction*. New York: Harper and Row.

Green, B. S. 1995. *Jogging the Mind: How to Use Aerobic Exercise as Meditation*. Dingman's Ferry, PA: Silverlake Press.

Greenberg, D., and C. A. Oglesby. 1997. Mental health dimensions. In *Physical Activity and Sport in the Lives of Girls: Physical and Mental Health Dimensions from an Interdisciplinary Approach*. Rockville, MD: SAMHSA.

Greist, J. H., M. H. Klein, R. R. Eischens, J. Faris, A. S. Gurman, and W. P. Morgan. 1979. Running as treatment for depression. *Comprehensive Psychiatry* 20:41-54.

Grilo, C. 1996. Treatment of obesity: An integrative model. In *Body Image, Eating Disorders, and Obesity: An Integrative Guide for Assessment and Treatment*, edited by J. K. Thompson. Washington, DC: American Psychological Association.

Hall, R. L. 1998. Softly strong: African American women's use of exercise in therapy. In *Integrating Exercise, Sports, Movement, and Mind: Therapeutic Unity*, edited by K. F. Hays. Binghamton, NY: Haworth.

Hays, K. F. 1994. Running therapy: Special characteristics and therapeutic issues of concern. *Psychotherapy* 31:725-734.

———. 1999. *Working It Out: Using Exercise in Psychotherapy.* Washington, DC: APA.

Heil, J., and K. Henschen. 1996. Assessment in sport and exercise psychology. In *Exploring Sport and Exercise Psychology*, edited by J. L. Van Raalte and B. W. Brewer. Washington, DC: American Psychological Association.

Henschen, K. P. 1998. Athletic staleness and burnout: Diagnosis, prevention, and treatment. In *Applied Sport Psychology: Personal Growth to Peak Performance*, 3rd ed., edited by J. M. Williams. Mountain View, CA: Mayfield.

Holmes, D. S. 1993. Aerobic fitness and the response to psychological stress. In *Exercise Psychology: The Influence of Physical Exercise on Psychological Processes*, edited by P. Seraganian. New York: Wiley.

Horn, T. S., and R. P. Claytor. 1993. Developmental aspects of exercise psychology. In *Exercise Psychology: The Influence of Physical Exercise on Psychological Processes*, edited by P. Seraganian. New York: Wiley.

Johnsgard, K. W. 1989. *The Exercise Prescription for Depression and Anxiety.* New York: Plenum.

Kabat-Zinn, J. 1990. *Full Catastrophe Living.* New York: Dell.

Kahn, A. P., and J. Fawcett. 1993. *The Encyclopedia of Mental Health.* New York: Facts on File.

Kavussanu, M., and E. McAuley. 1995. Exercise and optimism: Are highly active individuals more optimistic? *Journal of Sport and Exercise Psychology* 17:246-258.

Khatri, P., J. A. Blumenthal, M. A. Babyak, W. E. Craighead, S. Herman, T. Baldewicz, D. J. Madden, M. Doraiswamy, R. Waugh, and K. R. Krishnan. 2001. Effects of exercise training on cognitive functioning among depressed older men and women. *Journal of Aging and Physical Activity* 9:43-57.

Kirschenbaum, D. S. 1992. Elements of effective weight control programs: Implications for exercise and sport psychology. *Journal of Applied Sport Psychology*, 4, 77-93.

———. 1994. *Weight Loss Through Persistence: Making Science Work for You.* Oakland, CA: New Harbinger.

Klein, M. H., J. H. Greist, A. S. Gurman, R. A. Neimeyer, D. P. Lesser, N. J. Bushnell, and R. E. Smith. 1985. A comparative outcome study of group psychotherapy vs. exercise treatments for depression. *International Journal of Mental Health* 13:148-177.

Koeppl, P. M., J. Heller, E. R. Bleecker, D. A. Meyers, A. P. Goldberg, and M. L. Bleecker. 1992. The influence of weight reduction and exercise regimes upon the personality profiles of overweight males. *Journal of Clinical Psychology* 48:463-471.

Kostrubala, T. 1977. *The Joy of Running.* New York: Pocket.

Kremer, D., M. J. Malkin, and J. J. Benshoff. 1995. Physical activity programs offered in substance abuse treatment facilities. *Journal of Substance Abuse Treatment* 12:327-333.

Kritz-Silverstein, D., E. Barrett-Connor, and C. Corbeau. 2001. Cross-sectional and prospective study of exercise and depressed mood in the elderly: The Rancho Bernardo study. *American Journal of Epidemiology* 153:596-603.

Krucoff, C., and M. Krucoff. 2000. *Healing Moves: How to Cure, Relieve, and Prevent Common Ailments with Exercise.* New York: Harmony.

Lake, N. 2001. Say amen to fitness. *The Walking Magazine*, June, 36-41.

Laurin, D., R. Verreault, J. Lindsay, K. MacPherson, and K. Rockwood. 2001. Physical activity and risk of cognitive impairment and dementia in elderly persons. *Archives of Neurology* 58:498-504.

Leith, L. M. 1994. *Foundations of Exercise and Mental Health*. Morgantown, WV: Fitness Information Technology.

Long, B. C. 1985. Stress-management interventions: A 15-month follow-up of aerobic conditioning and stress inoculation training. *Cognitive Therapy and Research* 9:471-478.

Long, B. C., and C. J. Haney. 1988. Long-term follow-up of stressed working women: A comparison of aerobic exercise and progressive relaxation. *Journal of Sport and Exercise Psychology* 10:461-470.

Martinsen, E. W. 1990. Benefits of exercise for the treatment of depression. *Sports Medicine* 9:380-389.

Martinsen, E. W., and W. P. Morgan. 1997. Antidepressant effects of physical activity. In *Physical Activity and Mental Health*, edited by W. P. Morgan. Washington, DC: Taylor and Francis.

McCann, S. 1995. Overtraining and burnout. In *Sport Psychology Interventions*, edited by S. M. Murphy. Champaign, IL: Human Kinetics.

McCann, L., and D. S. Holmes. 1984. Influence of aerobic exercise on depression. *Journal of Personality and Social Psychology* 46:1142-1147.

McDonald, D. G., and J. A. Hodgdon. 1991. *The Psychological Effects of Aerobic Fitness Training: Research and Theory*. New York: Springer-Verlag.

McGrath, E., G. P. Keita, B. R. Strickland, and N. F. Russo. 1990. *Women and Depression*. Washington, DC: American Psychological Association.

Miller, W. R., and S. A. Brown. 1997. Why psychologists should treat alcohol and drug problems. *American Psychologist* 52: 1269-1279.

Mondin, G. W., W. P. Morgan, P. N. Piering, A. J. Stegner, C. L. Stotesbery, M. R. Trine, and M. Y. Wu. 1996. Psychological consequences of exercise deprivation in habitual exercisers. *Medicine and Science in Sports and Exercise* 28:1199-1203.

Morgan, W. P., ed. 1997. *Physical Activity and Mental Health*. Washington, DC: Taylor and Francis.

Morgan, W. P., D. L. Costill, M. G. Flynn, J. S. Raglin, and P. J. O'Connor. 1988. Mood disturbance following increased training in swimmers. *Medicine and Science in Sports and Exercise* 20:408-414.

Murphy, M., and R. A. White. 1995. *In the zone* (Rev. ed.). New York: Penguin.

Murphy, S. M. 1996. *The Achievement Zone*. New York: Putnam's.

Murphy, T. J., R. R. Pagano, and G. A. Marlatt. 1986. Lifestyle modification with heavy alcohol drinkers: Effects of aerobic exercise and meditation. *Addictive Behaviors* 11:175-186.

Nhat Hanh, T. 1992. *Peace Is Every Step*. New York: Bantam.

North, T. C., P. McCullagh, and Z. V. Tran. 1990. Effect of exercise on depression. *Exercise and Sport Sciences Reviews* 18:379-415.

O'Connor, P. J., J. C. Smith, and W. P. Morgan. 2000. Physical activity does not provoke panic attacks in patients with panic disorder: A review of the evidence. *Anxiety, Stress, and Coping* 13:333-353.

One in five Americans depressed or unhappy. 2000. *Reuters Health* November 8.

Orwin, A. 1973. "The running treatment": A preliminary communication on a new use for an old therapy (physical activity) in the agoraphobic syndrome. *British Journal of Psychiatry* 122:175-179.

Paffenbarger, R. S. and E. Olsen. 1996. *Lifefit: an Effective Exercise Program for Optimal Health and a Longer Life.* Champaign, IL: Human Kinetics.

Physical activity & sport in the lives of girls: Physical and mental health dimensions from an interdisciplinary approach. 1997. Rockville, MD: SAMHSA.

Pincus, H. A., T. L. Tanielian, S. C. Marcus, M. Olfson, D. A. Zarin, J. Thompson, and J. M. Zito. 1998. Prescribing trends in psychotropic medications: Primary care, psychiatry, and other medical specialties. *Journal of the American Medical Association* 279:526-531.

Powers, J. M., G. E. Woody, and M. L. Sachs. 1999. Perceived effects of exercise and sport in a population defined by their injection drug use. *American Journal on Addictions* 8: 71-75.

Prior, J. C., K. Gill, & Y. M. Vigna. 1995. Fluoxetine for premenstrual dysphoria. *New England Journal of Medicine* 333:1152.

Prochaska, J. O. 1996. *A Revolution in Health Promotion: How Unhealthy Lifestyles Can Be Changed.* Paper presented at Frontiers of Knowledge, Concord, New Hampshire. November.

Prochaska, J. O., and B. H. Marcus. 1994. The transtheoretical model: Applications to exercise. In *Advances in Exercise Adherence*, edited by R. K. Dishman. Champaign, IL: Human Kinetics.

Prochaska, J. O., J. C. Norcross, and C. C. DiClemente. 1994. *Changing for Good.* New York: William Morrow.

Progoff, I. 1975. *At a Journal Workshop.* New York: Dialogue House Library.

Raglin, J. S. 1993. Overtraining and staleness: Psychometric monitoring of endurance athletes. In *Handbook of Research on Sport Psychology*, edited by R. B. Singer, M. Murphey, and L. K. Tennant. New York: Macmillan.

———. 1997. Anxiolytic effects of physical activity. In *Physical Activity and Mental Health*, edited by W. P. Morgan. Washington, DC: Taylor and Francis.

Rejeski, W. J., and A. Thompson. 1993. Historical and conceptual roots of exercise psychology. In *Exercise Psychology: The Influence of Physical Exercise on Psychological Processes*, edited by P. Seraganian. New York: Wiley.

Rindskopf, K. D., and S. E. Gratch. 1982. Women and exercise: A therapeutic approach. *Women and Therapy* 1:15-26.

Rich, F. 1997. Journal: Harnisch's perfect pitch. *New York Times*, May 1, A27.

Rodin, J. 1992. *Body Traps: Breaking the Binds That Keep You from Feeling Good about Your Body*. New York: Quill.

Rodin, J., L. R. Silberstein, and R. H. Striegel-Moore. 1984. Women and weight: A normative discontent. In *Nebraska Symposium on Motivation: Psychology and Gender*, vol. 32, edited by T. B. Sonderegger. Lincoln, NE: University of Nebraska Press.

Sachs, M. L. 1984. The mind of the runner: Cognitive strategies used during running. In *Running as Therapy: An Integrated Approach*, edited by M. L. Sachs and G. W. Buffone. Lincoln, NE: University of Nebraska Press.

Sacks, O. 1997. Water babies: Why I love to swim. *The New Yorker*, May 26, 44-45.

Sallis, J. F., B. G. Simons-Morton, E. J. Stone, C. B. Corbin, L. H. Epstein, N. Faucette, R. J. Iannotti, J. D. Killen, R. C. Klesges, C. K. Petray, T. W. Rowland, and W. C. Taylor. 1992. Determinants of physical activity and interventions in youth. *Medicine and Science in Sports and Exercise* 24:S192-S195.

SAMHSA. 1997. *Physical Activity and Sport in the Lives of Girls: Physical and Mental Health Dimensions from an Interdisciplinary Approach*. 1997. Rockville, MD: SAMHSA.

Seligman, M. E. P. 1991. *Learned Optimism*. New York: Knopf.

Seligman, M. E. P., and M. Csikszentmihalyi. 2000. Positive psychology: An introduction. *American Psychologist* 55:5-14.

Seraganian, P. 1993. Current status and future directions in the field of exercise psychology. In *Exercise Psychology: The Influence of Physical Exercise on Psychological Processes*, edited by P. Seraganian. New York: Wiley.

Selye, H. 1975. *Stress Without Distress*. New York: Signet.

Sheehan, G. 1978. *Running and Being: The Total Experience*. New York: Warner Books.

———. 1996. *Going the Distance: One Man's Journey to the End of His Life*. New York: Villard.

Sime, W. E. 1996. Guidelines for clinical applications of exercise therapy for mental health. In *Exploring Sport and Exercise Psychology*, edited by J. L. Van Raalte and B. W. Brewer. Washington, DC: American Psychological Association.

Sinyor, D., T. Brown, L. Rostant, and P. Seraganian. 1982. The role of a physical fitness program in the treatment of alcoholism. *Journal of Studies on Alcohol* 43:380-386.

Sonstroem, R. J. 1997. Physical activity and self-esteem. In *Physical Activity and Mental Health*, edited by W. P. Morgan. Washington, DC: Taylor and Francis.

Steege, J. F., and J. A. Blumenthal. 1993. The effects of aerobic exercise on premenstrual symptoms in middle-aged women: A preliminary study. *Journal of Psychosomatic Research* 37:127-133.

Stephenson, M. G., A. S. Levy, M. L. Sass, and W. E. McGarvey. 1987. 1985 NHIS findings: Nutrition knowledge and baseline data for the weight-loss objectives. *Public Health Report* 102:61-67.

Steptoe, A., J. Moses, S. Edwards, and A. Mathews. 1993. Exercise and responsivity to mental stress: Discrepancies between the subjective and physiological effects of aerobic training. *International Journal of Sport Psychology* 24:110-129.

Striegel-Moore, R. H., L. R. Silberstein, and J. Rodin. 1986. Toward an understanding of risk factors for bulimia. *American Psychologist* 41:246-263.

Thayer, R. E., J. R. Newman, and T. M. McClain. 1994. Self-regulation of mood: Strategies for changing a bad mood, raising energy, and reducing tension. *Journal of Personality and Social Psychology* 67:910-925.

The Walking Magazine. 2001. June.

Theriault, D., D. Richard, A. Labrie, and G. Theriault. 1997. Physiological and psychological variables in swimmers during a competitive season in relation to the overtraining syndrome. *Medicine and Science in Sports and Exercise* [Supplement abstract] 29(5):1237.

Thompson, R. A., and R. T. Sherman. 1993. *Helping Athletes with Eating Disorders*. Champaign, IL: Human Kinetics.

Too few people are treated for depression. 1997. *APA Monitor*, March, 6.

Ullyot, J. 1976. *Women Running*. Mountain View, CA: World Publications.

United States Department of Health and Human Services. 1996. *Physical Activity and Health: A Report of the Surgeon General*. Atlanta, GA: U.S. Department of Health and Human Services, Centers for Disease Control and Prevention, National Center for Chronic Disease Prevention and Health Promotion.

U.S. News and World Report, January 22, 2001.

Wallace, L.S., J. Buckworth, T. E. Kirby, & W. M. Sherman. 2000. Characteristics of exercise behavior among college students: Application of social cognitive theory to predicting stage of change. *Journal of Preventive Medicine* 31:494-505.

Walsh, B. T., and D. M. Garner. 1997. Diagnostic issues. In *Handbook of Treatment for Eating Disorders*, 2nd ed., edited by D. M. Garner and P. E. Garfinkel. New York: Guilford.

Wankel, L. M. 1993. The importance of enjoyment to adherence and psychological benefits from physical activity. *International Journal of Sport Psychology* 24:151-169.

Whiston, S. C., and T. L. Sexton. 1993. An overview of psychotherapy outcome research: Implications for practice. *Professional Psychology: Research and Practice* 24:43-51.

Wiese-Bjornstal, D. 1997. Psychological dimensions. In *Physical Activity and Sport in the Lives of Girls: Physical and Mental Health Dimensions from an Interdisciplinary Approach*. Rockville, MD: SAMHSA.

Yates, A. 1991. *Compulsive Exercise and the Eating Disorders: Toward an Integrated Theory of Activity*. New York: Brunner-Mazel.

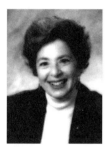 **Kate Hays, Ph.D.**, is the president of the sport psychology division of the American Psychological Association. She has been practicing psychology for over 25 years, in New Hampshire and Toronto. Support for her clients' use of exercise as one aspect of their mental well-being is a regular aspect of her practice. Dr. Hays is active as both a Fellow of the American Psychological Association and a Fellow and Certified Consultant of the Association for the Advancement of Applied Sport Psychology.

She is also the author of *Working It Out: Using Exercise in Psychotherapy* and *Integrating Exercise, Sports, Movement and Mind: Therapeutic Unity*.